Gary Marks –

Bob Lilley –

Culture of

CW00616444

Forensic Phonetics

Forensic Phonetics

John Baldwin and *Peter French*

Pinter Publishers
London and New York

© John Baldwin and Peter French 1990

First published in Great Britain in 1990 by
Pinter Publishers Limited
25 Floral Street, London WC2E 9DS

British Library Cataloguing in Publication Data

A CIP catalogue record for this book is available from the
British Library
ISBN 0 86187 786 1

For enquiries in North America please contact PO Box 197, Irvington,
NY 10553

Library of Congress Cataloging-in-Publication Data

Baldwin, John R.
    Forensic phonetics / by John Baldwin and Peter French.
        p. cm.
    Includes bibliographical references (p.   ).
    ISBN 0-86187-786-1
    1. Criminal investigation. 2. Phonetics. I. French, Peter.
II. Title.
HV8073.B343   1990   90-35038
363.2'58—dc20   CIP

Filmset by Mayhew Typesetting, Bristol, UK
Printed in Great Britain by
Billing & Sons Ltd, Worcester

Contents

Foreword

This book is the outcome of a casual and fortuitous conversation over lunch a few years ago between John Baldwin and Robin Fawcett, editor of the 'Open Linguistics Series' for Pinter Publishers Ltd. Robin followed up a vague agreement at the time with a firm proposal for a book on Forensic Phonetics which John, after some cogitation, accepted. As the writing proceeded, however, it became increasingly clear that the general scope of it would take it outside the area originally intended. It would, of course, still have to deal with phonetics, but it seemed that this could best be presented and discussed in the wider context of actual forensic cases. There is, too, some discussion of the psychology of certain types of criminal and of transcript-writers, as well as the airing of several contentious issues in the matter of speaker-identification by means of phonetic comparison. A further, and major topic is the adversarial system in English criminal law.

All of these issues are introduced by the present writers in the first person singular; 'I' refers to John Baldwin everywhere but in Chapter 3 – Acoustics, which was written by Peter French. Readers will soon discover that there are certain matters on which the writers do not see eye to eye. We are not disturbed by such disagreements, but, on the contrary, consider them in this area to be both inevitable and natural. We believe that, by approaching them in a rational and positive manner, we will be able to contribute in a productive way to developments in the area of forensic phonetics.

John Baldwin   Peter French
London   York

List of symbols

The following are phonemic symbols for English Received Pronunciation (RP).

Vowels and diphthongs

1.	/iː	*fleece, bean, see*
2.	ɪ	*kit, dig, city*
3.	e	*dress, red*
4.	æ	*trap, glad*
5.	aː	*start, palm, bath, car*
6.	ɒ	*lot, dog, cloth*
7.	ɔː	*thought, born, four, jaw*
8.	ʊ	*foot, put good*
9.	uː	*goose, food, true*
10.	ʌ	*strut, love*
11.	ɜː	*nurse, burn, stir*
12. (schwa)	ə	another
13.	eɪ	face, main, bay
14.	əʊ	goat, own, no
15.	aɪ	price, time, buy
16.	aʊ	mouth, loud, now
17.	ɔɪ	choice, void, boy
18.	ɪə	near, beard, idea
19.	eə	*square, scarce, pair*
20.	ʊə/	*cure, (poor)*

Consonants

/p	pin	b	bin
t	tin	d	din
k	come	g	gum
tʃ	chain	dʒ	Jane
f	fine	v	vine
θ	think	ð	this
s	seal	z	zeal
ʃ	sheep	ʒ	measure
h	how		
m	sum	l	light
n	sun	r	right
ŋ	sung	j	yet
		w/	wet

Chapter 1

Introduction

In this Introduction I propose to deal with a number of important matters which lie within the legal domain on the one hand, and in the phonetics domain on the other. All of these matters are relevant to forensic phonetics as such, and I think an examination of them now will provide a vital background to the descriptions of cases and discussions of principles to be found later in the book. Some of the points to be discussed below are highly contentious, and I hope that readers, whatever their own specialised areas of activity, will gain some helpful insights into the kinds of issues which exercise forensic phoneticians. It is conceivable, too, that the reader whose own background is in neither the law nor phonetics will find something of interest to them here, whether it be in these particular issues or in the general business of applying phonetics in the forensic field.

Fortunately, not everything is contentious; I would not, for example, expect any adverse comment from the academic world on a working definition of 'phonetics' as the art/science of the description of the sounds of speech. This definition, though laconic, will serve our purpose in the present chapter, and any deficiencies in it will be remedied in full in Chapter 2. If we read about the nature of speech in books on phonetics we will be informed that speech is elusive and that it presents special difficulties to the analyser. Phonetics in this aspect is a highly practical subject, and we do not, therefore, have to rely on what books tell us, useful though that may be. If we wish to, we can put the matter to the test ourselves, by introspecting on any speech act; there is little doubt that we will confirm that speech is indeed most elusive. It is a common experience that the more one tries to focus on speech in order to observe what is happening, the more it seems to change, to slip out of focus. There are a number of reasons for this, the first and most obvious being that a speech act - an utterance in other words - is transient, leaving no visible traces in the environment. Any examination of the phonetic substance as opposed to the meaning of an utterance will depend, if that utterance has not been electronically or otherwise recorded, on our auditory memory. We can certainly remember quite a lot of things about an utterance that we have just heard: for example, we would probably notice if there had been any marked speech defect, and perhaps a regional accent might impinge on our awareness under certain circumstances. Any prominent indicator of state of health, such as a blocked nose or hoarse voice would, too, be potentially retained in the memory. There is, however, a strict limit to the amount of detail about the phonetic substance of an utterance that can be remembered even under the most favourable of circumstances, because, after all, our attention is devoted primarily to extracting the relevant message for us in the utterance. It can happen only rarely that all the phonetic details of an utterance constitute part of its message, and in such a way that we are able to recapture those details in our auditory memories. A possible example of this would be when a speaker produces the word 'Yes' in a drawn-out manner, on a relatively low pitch, with a pitch-movement that falls and then rises, and with the lips slightly pursed in order to express agreement of the most grudging and sceptical kind. It seems also to be the case that people exhibit considerably variability in the efficiency of their auditory memories; however, there are so many unknown factors involved here that I believe it is true to say that there is no way in which the efficiency of the auditory memory of any given individual can be explained, let alone predicted.

Speech can be recorded on tape, allowing us repeated access to selected sections of it, but, far from making things easier, this only introduces further complications, particularly in the form of the extreme variability of speech. This is almost certain to exceed, and by a considerable measure, anything that our auditory memories could encompass on a single hearing. For example, if we listen to a number of repetitions of the 'same' word by the same speaker, we are very likely to discover that every such repetition sounds slightly, or even markedly different. This is because of a very large number of variables, the most obvious of which are changes in the pitch of the voice, i.e. the musical note(s) on which the utterance is produced, changes in the tempo of the utterance, changes in the voice quality (see Chapter 2), changes in the ways in which the vowels and consonants themselves are produced, and so on and so on. This is by no means an exhaustive list of variables, and if we add to it those of the preceding paragraph relating to states of the speaker's health, we arrive at what we might perceive as a very disturbing picture of the nature of speech - something so fraught with variation that it would seem very difficult to say anything sensible about it at all! And if we consider it from the forensic point of view, where samples of speech could possibly need to be compared for the purposes of speaker-identification, the prospects of our ever getting samples which would permit meaningful comparison might seem even more remote.

Amongst academic phoneticians there are some who do take this, what I will call 'negativist' view of the forensic application of phonetics to the matter of speaker-identification; they are acutely aware of the seemingly infinite variability of speech that I have tried to depict above, and conclude that, indeed, no reliable comparison *can* be made of speech samples in the forensic context. The negativists divide, I believe, into two camps: firstly, those who believe that nothing of any validity can be said when speech samples are to be compared. These ultra-negativists would not, for example, be prepared to give an opinion as to whether two speech samples *might* have been spoken by the same person; nor would they offer any view that two given samples were *not* spoken by the same person. This at least seems logical to me, even though I do not subscribe to such an attitude, because if one starts from the premise of infinite and arbitrary variability in speech, then it does indeed follow that nothing whatsoever can be said about it forensically.

The second group of negativists, who might perhaps, and without offence, be designated the 'wets' as opposed to the 'ultra's', are those who would never accept that two speech samples can be shown by their phonetic similarity to have been produced by the same person, even to a low level of probability, but would consider it academically valid to eliminate speakers, i.e. to establish negative identifications on the basis of phonetic differences. It has certainly been my experience that it is easier to arrive at negative identifications than at positive ones, for reasons to be discussed later (Chapter 4), but I am unable to perceive the logic of the position that affords validity only to negative, but not to positive comparisons. For reasons which should become clear very shortly, I believe that phonetic comparison in the forensic context must either be accepted or rejected, and that the middle ground is untenable.

Some academic phoneticians do not operate in the forensic area because they simply do not have time to take on more work, whilst others when asked say that they do not wish to get involved. In the latter instance this is presumably because of the kinds of case and/or the kinds of people that they find, or suppose they would find, distasteful if they were involved with them. I respect these positions, of course; as far as the second goes, there are certainly both people and cases I have encountered that could most adequately be described in that way. It is a matter for regret, though, that more phoneticians are not willing to undertake forensic work, especially at the present time where there seems to be a greatly expanding field of opportunity. In many areas of the legal system the help of professional phoneticians is becoming more and more urgently needed; if they are not prepared to come forward, there are, unfortunately, numbers of other putative experts with minimal or non-existent phonetic sophistication who are ready enough to fill the vacuum.

If we now consider the 'positivists', we discover a comparable range of opinions to those examined above in relation to the 'negativists'. Positivists have in common the belief that comparisons of speech samples for forensic purposes are acceptable, and that they can produce both positive and negative identifications. It is at this point that unanimity ceases. It is, I think, of interest to note in passing that the positivist tradition is very strongly established in some universities, whereas in others negativism seems to predominate. For example, as far as I am aware, the positivist tradition at University College London was initiated in the early 1960s by the then Professor of Experimental Phonetics, Dennis Fry, who was involved in a number of civil and criminal cases. That tradition continues now, even though relatively few of my colleagues undertake forensic work. In other universities, such as Leeds, a fairly recent tradition of negativism prevails, with certain notable exceptions. I think it is probably true to say, too, that many, perhaps even most phoneticians would prefer not to take up any particular position in this argument.

Historically speaking, the first positive approach to speaker-identification was of a purely acoustic character. It was believed that measurement of the sound waves of speech by electronic devices, principally the sound-spectrograph, could produce print-outs which would be the speech equivalent of finger-prints – the so-called 'voice-prints' that everyone seems to have heard of. This matter is dealt with in some detail in the chapter by Peter French (Chapter 3), and will also be returned to in the final chapter of the book, in which future prospects are discussed. It will, therefore, suffice at this point to say that such an approach was soon shown to be ineffective. At this time, as far as I am aware, no one in the British Isles who knows anything about the complexity of speech, certainly no professional phonetician, would consider using such a method for forensic purposes. When it is used thus, it seems to be by people qualified in other areas whose understanding of the problems which arise from the variability of speech is both lamentably and dangerously naive.

Another school of positivists places sole reliance in the auditory approach, i.e. in the effectiveness of the human ear alone. Those subscribing to this view, and that includes the present writer, are fully aware of the speech-variability problem, indeed, they may well have had more experience in listening to and analysing samples of natural speech than the negativists, but do not accept their conclusion that that problem must of necessity render the phonetician impotent in the matter of forensic comparison. They would point out that the phrase: 'the human ear alone' is actually rather misleading, since it is impossible for the human ear to function without involving the human brain. The phrase must, therefore, be understood to include the inevitable back-up of the human brain. Even the most advanced electronic devices, linked with the most power-ful computers, have no built-in facility for the interpretation of the measurements they make (and it is a matter of the greatest difficulty to program them to do so), but the human brain, on the other hand, is uniquely equipped to do precisely that. Inter-pretation by the 'human computer' of the apparent chaos of variability in speech reduces it to order by filtering out what is not relevant in a particular situation, and renders speech amenable both to principled description and comparison. Human interpretation, then, is always going to be essential in no matter what area of speech study one is involved; it is, indeed, probably true of any field of study – it is never possible simply to switch on the machines and leave them both to make measurements and to interpret the measurements they have made.

To revert to an earlier point: if interpretation in this sense is acceptable in producing negative identifications, as it seems to be to some negativists, then it is difficult, to say the least, to understand their rejection of those same processes in the case of positive identifications. The point is that when we listen, as phoneticians, to speech samples and compare them, we are naturally going to observe many more phonetic features than the layman could. Any conclusions as to the 'sameness' or 'differentness' of those samples must depend on the judgement of the phonetician, his internal processing of that complex material, since he cannot refer to any external, experimentally-based criteria to help him decide what is significant and what is not.

By way of a slight digression: the human brain in some circumstances could be considered to be too powerful, i.e. when one of its functions interferes with another of its functions. This is experienced when objective perception of speech is influenced by preconceived ideas held in the brain about what kinds of things can happen in speech. For example, our first reaction to the sounds of a foreign language is to interpret them in terms of our own language; indeed, if we are not linguistically talented to any extent, that will remain our only reaction, no matter how long we are in contact with that foreign language. I am sure every reader will know someone to whom that description applies! With proper training and the necessary motivation, however, anyone with a modicum of ability can make drastic improvements in their pronunciation of even the most difficult of foreign languages.

As discussed later (Chapter 2), the auditory phonetic description of sounds requires objectivity on the part of the describer. Students of phonetics, too, begin with the familiar layman's reactions to novel sounds - as when they describe a 'voiced bilabial fricative' as: 'a funny sort of "b"' or a 'rounded front close-mid vowel' as: 'a funny sort of "er"', and so on (see Chapter 2 for explanations and symbols). Clearly their brains are not accepting as 'real' the unfamiliar sounds, and must be persuaded to do so; this is usually successfully achieved by the application of trusted and long-established training techniques on the part of teachers of phonetics.

In the forensic context there is the ever-present danger that the phonetics expert's conclusions as to the 'sameness' or 'differentness' of the samples he is comparing could be influenced by his previously acquired beliefs about the subjects involved. The possibility exists, and it is not purely theoretical, that he could be influenced by the expectations of those consulting him. This danger is particularly great when, as is usually the case of course, he is consulted by either prosecution or defence. In the past it quite often happened to me, as well as to some of my colleagues, that there was a determined and not very subtle attempt by one or more members of the relevant 'team' to influence my conclusions. This was usually done either by listing the various iniquities of the accused: 'beats his wife, suspected of complicity in all manner of unsavoury dealings, drinks', etc., etc., obviously a true enemy of society deserving to be brought to book, on the part of the prosecution, or depicting him as: 'a pillar of the community, honest and blameless in every aspect of his existence, sober', etc., etc., clearly a prospective candidate for beatification, on the part of the defence. It is many years now since anyone has tried to influence me in that way, perhaps because I have stopped looking so gullible, or, rather more likely I hope, that it is no longer seen as proper behaviour towards an expert who is, in both principle and practice, independent. The palpable inappropriateness of the dichotomy of prosecution and defence with regard to the expert, whether phonetics expert or otherwise, will be a recurrent theme of this book.

Returning now to the subject of the use of electronic devices for analysing speech in the forensic context – a topic we departed from a few paragraphs ago – we must consider the third approach to speaker-identification: the method which combines the auditory with the acoustic. Here analyses are made by both means, and the results of the auditory approach cross-checked against the instrumental print-outs. The implication often is that the auditory judgments are likely to be less sound than the electronic ones, and that the latter represent a 'scientifically-based' means of discovering whether the auditory judgments are right or not. This, again, implies that the acoustic measurements represent a higher level of analysis, a greater degree of objectivity, such that they have the status of a reference point against which auditorily-made judgments are to be compared; if they are found to be different, the auditory judgments must be rejected in favour of the allegedly higher reality of the acoustic measurements.

One psychological explanation for the primacy which is

accorded the acoustic analysis is that it is available in the visual form of a print-out from a machine. It is common knowledge that our visual sense is far more evolved than our auditory sense, and this explains the instinct of the layman, but not only the layman, to put his trust more happily in visual forms than in auditory forms. The reality of the matter is, though, that speech analysis carried out by electronic devices is simply another way of analysing speech, not representing a higher level of reality which is superior to auditory analysis, but presenting its own advantages and, most importantly, its own disadvantages. As one might expect, these are usually problems arising from the unavoidable requirement of interpretation. I would argue that acoustic analysis is of equal value to auditory analysis, and that both methods are, of necessity, imperfect – both rely on interpretation and both, as human activities, are therefore susceptible to error. I am sure that no phonetician, no matter what his approach to speaker-identification, would claim infallibility for his method. I would certainly not wish to raise any objection to the combined acoustic/auditory approach, so long as it retained the principle of equal status that I have been arguing for above. I would, however, contest most strongly any suggestion of the primacy of acoustic analysis. It is my experience that the auditory approach can stand alone, whereas the acoustic approach cannot, and this seems to represent the true state of things.

A number of forensic phoneticians, though I am not among them, for reasons that I shall come to shortly, present aspects of their evidence in court by means of spectrograms, and so on. I believe that this is done as visual back-up to the auditory evidence, i.e. confirmation of conclusions arrived at auditorily and visual presentation of those conclusions for the convenience of the court. It is not, if I understand their position correctly, that they are claiming a higher status for such evidence, simply that it gets their point across to the court in a more effective way. I have no wish to criticise that practice. In presenting my own evidence in court I have not found it necessary to make use of visual means in the form we are speaking of. It has been my experience in something like thirty appearances, both before magistrates, juries and tribunals, that auditorily-based evidence can be perfectly well explained in its own terms, without recourse to other forms of presentation. I would, too, be unwilling to run the risk of giving the court the

impression, however vaguely, that I had used the auditory/
acoustic approach when in fact I had not.

The reader will have gathered that there is a certain amount
of disagreement in the academic world at the present time as to
which method should be employed in forensics, and I will
summarise my position on that matter by saying that I have
found the auditory approach to be fully adequate for the task. I
would accept the auditory/acoustic approach as helpful, so long
as the balance were inclined to the auditory. Neither method is
perfect, of course, in the sense that both include the possibility
of error; they are, however, the best we have at this time. With
regard to the different kinds of negativism discussed above, I
believe my attitude to them can be perceived unequivocably
enough, and I shall, therefore, say nothing further. Given the
present state of the art, I do not think that voice-prints are
technically possible yet, although future developments could be
interesting (Chapter 6).

The attractiveness of voice-prints, if they existed, would lie in
their potential for offering identification, whether positive or
negative, in a categorical manner; like finger-prints they could
give 100 per cent conclusions. In the case of forensic phonetics,
though, one is never dealing with such a level of certainty. All
conclusions in this area must be stated by the phonetician as
opinions, just as handwriting, medical and other experts are
accustomed to doing. The very use of the word 'opinion' entails
an element of doubt, a possibility of error which is present in
all human activities. The forensic phonetician reaches his
conclusions on the basis of his own analyses of the material he
has examined, and both the procedures and the conclusions are
expressed in terms which are meaningful to other phoneticians
(to be dealt with more fully at a later point). Those conclusions,
being based on human perceptions, are of necessity phrased in
terms of imprecise categories rather than as percentages. There
was a brief period many years ago when I presented my opinions
as percentages in one or two cases, but I realised that by so
doing I was giving the court a misleading impression of
accuracy, since I could not adduce figures in support of those
final percentages. I abandoned that practice in favour of what
might appear the weaker position of using imprecise categories.
In fact, the apparently weaker position is stronger, for example
when attacked under cross-examination, because it is founded
on a realistic assessment of the nature of speech. If it were

possible to assign numerical values to the phonetic features of
speech, such as by rating vowel and consonant similarities on
a scale from zero to ten, such precise figures would be feasible.
However, as will be made adequately clear in Chapter 2
(Phonetics), the complexity of speech means that any such
attempt will be doomed to failure. Given that auditory
judgments are by their nature imprecise, in the mathematical
sense, it is appropriate that the categories in which they are
presented in court should be correspondingly imprecise. Different phoneticians have different categories at the present time,
although there is some promise that uniform categories and
their labelling will be adopted in the not too distant future. The
set of categories with which I currently operate are:

positive identification
- 'sure beyond reasonable doubt'
- 'there can be very little doubt'
- 'highly likely'
- 'likely'
- 'very probable'
- 'probable'
- 'quite possible'
- 'possible' . . . that they are the same person.

negative identification
- 'probable'
- 'quite probable'
- 'likely'
- 'highly likely' . . . that they are different people.

I think the first item of my 'positive' set may need some
explanation. I use this when I have come to the most definite
position that I could come to, on the basis of very good samples
and in the presence of similarities in every aspect of comparison. I am as sure as I can be that the two people are the
same, but, of course, it must never be forgotten that I am stating
this as my opinion, with everything that entails.

In the early days, certainly in the 1960s, when tape-recording
was a relatively new and unfamiliar technology, it was a matter
of genuine uncertainty as to whether tape-recorded evidence
would be permitted by any given judge in any given trial. I
believe there were cases where such evidence was excluded by
the judge solely because it was tape-recorded, and there may

have been others where defence successfully argued against
acceptance of tape-recordings because they had been made
covertly, a point to which I shall return later (Chapter 4).
However, as far as my own cases are concerned, when such
evidence has been excluded, it has been for quite different
reasons. I should add that it is my impression that such exclu-
sion happens very rarely.

One case, heard in Northampton Crown Court, in which tape-
recorded evidence was rejected by the judge was that of T, a
young woman accused of having made a large number of hoax
telephone calls to the fire service, a local department store, a
factory, and so on. On some occasions the hoaxer claimed that
a bomb had been left on the premises, with all the inconvenience that entailed. On other occasions she reported fires which
did not exist. Whoever she was, she was causing a vast loss of
money in the form of wasted journeys by the fire service and
disruption of work when businesses were evacuated unneces-
sarily. It was clearly a matter of the greatest importance that
she should be identified and stopped.

A suspect was eventually brought in for interview. She was
someone who had a record of making such nuisance calls, and
the interview which the police conducted with her was
recorded. A copy of that recorded interview was sent to me so
that I could compare it with copies of the recordings of some of
the hoax telephone calls.

I should point out before going any further that it is
customary for phoneticians to use only first-generation copies,
i.e. not copies of copies, of original tape-recordings. There are a
few exceptions to that general pattern. One of them occurs
when the original recording has been made on a multi-track
drum recorder, such as is used by the public services to record
their incoming calls. It would clearly be extremely difficult,
since the drum is in constant use, for the person responsible for
making the copy tapes to produce a large number of copies
under those circumstances, especially when he does not know
for sure how many copies are eventually going to be needed. It
is clearly more practical for a single copy to be made as the
'master copy', and other copies to be made from this as and
when required. From the phoneticians' point of view it would
be extremely disquieting to have to take responsibility for
original evidence – if anything were to go wrong with the tapes
the consequences would not bear consideration. Doubts which

earlier were expressed in court by experts over the possibly deleterious effect of copying on a speech sample have evaporated with the advance of technology.

Another exception to the general principle that one only works with copies is when there are special reasons for not doing so. On only a handful of occasions have I been required to carry out my work on original recordings. These were sensitive cases in which copies were not permitted and in which I had to make my analyses and comparisons under police guard. Needless to say, I prefer not to have to work under those conditions!

Let us now return to the case of T. The samples were adequate for the purposes of analysis and comparison, as discussed fully in Chapter 4, and I came to the conclusion that T and the unknown female caller were, in fact, the same person. I submitted this opinion to the police, and in due course found myself waiting in the Crown court for the case to begin. I was told that defence counsel wished to contest the admissibility of the tape-recordings as evidence. This was a matter of some considerable importance to the prosecution, as their case relied almost entirely on those tapes. A trial-within-a-trial was ordered for the purpose of hearing legal arguments and the evidence of witnesses in the absence of the jury. I had just begun to repeat the standard Church of England oath: 'I swear by Almighty God that the evidence I shall give shall be the truth, the whole truth, and nothing but the truth', when proceedings were interrupted by defence counsel. Having asked the court's pardon for his interruption, he explained that he had done so because the wrong oath was being taken. There was, he said, a different oath to be taken in the case of a trial-within-a-trial, and should not that be administered? The judge, together with the rest of the court, looked extremely doubtful about the correctness of that statement, and there was much rummaging in legal tomes throughout. Then, from a number of quarters arose the single expression: 'He's right'. The correct oath was then duly administered and the hearing proceeded. Neither before nor since have I been asked to take a different oath under those circumstances, and there seems now to be only the single C. of E. oath given above. The thought has crossed my mind on a number of occasions that perhaps all those hearings in which the 'wrong' oath was sworn in a trial-within-a-trial could be declared mistrials, but I have shrunk from the implications of that.

Defence counsel presented two submissions to the court,

1. The jury must not be permitted to hear any material which could be prejudicial to the defendant.
2. If an expert witness is to give evidence, the jury must be given access to all the material that expert has used in order to come to his conclusions.

On the first submission there was, of course, no dissent, because that principle has long been enshrined in our legal system. In the case of T this was a real issue, because she had mentioned her previous convictions during her interview with the police. The interview tape could not, therefore, be played in its entirety to the jury, because of those prejudicial passages. The police had not taken the precaution of obtaining a back-up sample, and I had not warned them that such a thing might be necessary, basically I suppose, because we had not foreseen the possibility that the interview tape might be ruled inadmissible. Everything depended on the judge's reaction to the second submission.

Counsel's argument was that the interview tape had to be considered as a single, indivisible entity. It was not possible, he claimed, to accept parts of it, and to exclude other parts, because if that were done, if the tape were edited, the jury would not, self-evidently, have access to all the material I had used in arriving at my opinion. Prosecution counsel made a valiant effort to counter that argument by suggesting that the tape could be edited because I had not needed the incriminating sections to reach a conclusion – I would have come to that same conclusion without them. It is, in my experience, usual practice to edit anything of an incriminating character from interview tapes when they are to be played to the jury, with the sole proviso that the expert has not needed that material. The argument put forward by prosecution counsel, then, is usually, almost invariably in fact, accepted by courts, but on that occasion it was not. The judge ruled that the interview tape was inadmissible because it could neither be played in toto nor edited. With that ruling the prosecution case was withdrawn.

In trying to work out why that particular judge made that particular, and unusual ruling on that particular occasion, I have only been able to explain it in terms of the events that morning in court. I believe that the judge must have been overawed and disconcerted by defence counsel's intervention on the matter of the correct oath to be sworn in the trial-within-a-trial, and that he allowed himself to be persuaded by him into making a decision which he might not have made on another occasion.

Another occasion on which tape-recorded evidence was ruled inadmissible by a judge was in a case in which I had been consulted by Her Majesty's Customs and Excise. The accused was alleged to have carried out a large number of fraudulent export deals in which he was believed to have made considerable illicit profits. There were substantial samples both of his speech and of the unknown person setting up a deal. I had found no differences between those samples, but had found very considerable similarities; my identification of the accused with that person was commensurately positive. There was other evidence, but my identification of the accused on the basis of those recordings was vital to the prosecution case.

Defence was contesting the validity of phonetic identification, and had called a negativist colleague from Leeds University. A trial-within-a-trial was once again held, though no special oath on this occasion, to allow the judge to reach his decision. After I had presented my evidence in the usual way, and my colleague had offered her views on that evidence, namely, that it should not be accepted by the court, the judge asked me if there was any possibility of the jury's being prejudiced by the speech samples. This is by no means a usual question, but it was relevant in the case under discussion. The accused was a German national, and had a very marked Bavarian accent. The judge was concerned lest the jury might simply register the fact that both samples involved some sort of German accent, and make their own identification on the principle that all Germans sound alike when they speak English. I explained that it would be my job to make it clear to the jury that individual speech characteristics were present, and that my identification had been based on them. The judge retired to ponder these arguments.

In due course he returned to give his rulings. Firstly, in the matter of the admissibility of identification evidence based on phonetic comparison, he would wish to take no position, and emphasised that his ruling could not be interpreted as rejection of such evidence. On the second matter, he still felt considerable doubt as to the jury's ability to listen to the speech samples in an unprejudiced way, and he therefore proposed to rule those samples inadmissible, on the grounds that the accused might

not be given a fair trial. This ruling effectively removed the
mainstay of the prosecution's case, and proceedings were
dropped.

There were particular circumstances in this case which, I
believed, tipped the balance for the judge in deciding whether
the samples were prejudicial or not. The accused, as I have
mentioned above, was a German national. That in itself was not
reason enough, but if we consider his disposition and
demeanour during the investigations and as heard on the admitted sample, we have at least part of the answer. He seemed to
embody every negative and unpleasant characteristic that could
be associated with Germans in English eyes. If someone had set
out to create a caricature of the worst kind of German
personality, they would have created the accused in this case!
Given that the trial judge was a Jew, I think we have the full
explanation. The judge, for good enough reason, was sensitive of
prejudice on many psychological levels, and was being more fair
than fair to the accused in, for all practical purposes, destroying
the prosecution case against him.

The playing of edited tapes in court is, as I have said, the rule
rather than the exception in my experience. Such editing is,
though, only accepted if it involves the presence of material
prejudicial to the defendant. Other material cannot be edited no
matter what its character, because of the requirement of con-
tinuity. Obviously, if tape-recorders were switched on and off
during, say, a meeting of men planning a crime, all manner of
allegations could be made about the periods which were not
recorded. The resulting unedited tapes can contain material
which proves to be rather embarrassing when played in court.
On one occasion I recall that a member of a gang planning to
carry out a robbery agreed with the police to carry a miniature
recording device on him when he went to the meeting with the
other gang members. He had been told how to switch the
recorder on, and that he should do so before leaving home for
the meeting. He had further been instructed that on no account
was he to switch the recorder off - come what may, he was to
leave it alone. When he reached the house in which the meeting
was to take place, he was overcome by an attack of diarrhoea,
conceivably as a result of his nervous condition due to his carrying the hidden recorder. He went straight to the lavatory in the
house, and faithfully refrained from turning off the recorder.
The ensuing events need not be described. In due course he

returned to the meeting, and everything went as planned, in that a good quality recording of that meeting was obtained which was subsequently used in a successful prosecution. The whole of this tape, though, had to be played in court, and, as one might suppose, varying degrees of embarrassment were evident! Colleagues have mentioned cases in which recordings of even more private events were played in open court, but both their examples and mine are, fortunately, rare. Whatever the topic of the speech he hears, the phonetician must ensure objectivity, and must treat it as, simply, material for analysis.

A number of terms to be used in the forthcoming pages should be defined at this point. These are not necessarily the same definitions to be found in the reference books, but rather those which I think will get the point across to the non-legal reader. The terms to be discussed here must be considered in their relationship to some of the characteristic features of English law. This is an adversarial system which, I believe, originates in the Anglo-Saxon custom of 'trial by combat'. One person would be accused of an offence, and both he and his accuser would fight it out in order to discover who was right. Such a custom must have been based on the belief that the Almighty would not allow a wrongdoer to triumph, and would assuredly, therefore, strengthen the arm of the righteous innocent. A very significant point to note here is that there does not appear to have been any very obvious requirement to find out the facts of the case. A further important point is that the whole objective of the operation was to win, because whoever won was clearly right, in the sight of the Lord. Modern English criminal law is a direct descendant of that earlier custom, but now the parties no longer fight it out themselves, and in the physical arena, but are represented by barristers: counsel for the prosecution and counsel for the defence, who fight their case verbally in a courtroom. The role of referee, presumably in the early cases acted by a tribal elder, has devolved upon the judges for some time now. Their basic function now as then is to ensure fair play – to see that everybody abides by the rules. I am aware that I may seem to have presented a very negative picture of English law here. It is one which, however regrettably, represents the truth of the underlying principles and attitudes as far as I have experienced them. I do not feel any doubt that our system is a bad one in many basic respects, which affords those who wish to obscure the truth and to win for the sake of winning full scope for those ambitions; I am equally convinced that most people operating in our system strive to see justice done, and the truth emerge. This topic will be discussed again in Chapter 6.

It would seem logical to begin with a consideration of what is meant by 'expert witness'. Such a witness is anyone with professional training and/or particular skills, such that he is able to express a specialist opinion on matters not within reach of the layman, i.e. the person not trained in that speciality. It is necessary to note the use of the word 'opinion' here. The expert witness is, in fact, the only kind of witness who can express an opinion as evidence, who, indeed, is expected to express an opinion. When a phonetician says that in his opinion two tape-recorded speech samples were made by the same person, that constitutes expert evidence, because he is giving the benefit of his training and experience. A police-officer who knows the suspect well, perhaps over several years, would usually be accepted by the court as an expert in that particular and specific respect, but this would not be likely to extend to an officer who has encountered the suspect for the first time in that recorded interview. Self-evidently, the expert's opinion is only 'expert' within the area of his training and experience; no professional phonetician would wish to go beyond that, of course, but instances are known of people claiming expertise in a remarkably wide range of subjects, and giving evidence in court on all of them.

In the nature of things, the expert is going to be talking about matters which will be unfamiliar to the jury; when his evidence is of a highly technical character, as in complex fraud cases, or the details of phonetic analysis (see Chapter 2, Phonetics), the jury will be able to understand very little concerning the facts themselves, and will be totally incapable of assessing the expert's interpretation of those facts. The obvious thing for the jury to do in that situation would be to work out as much as they can for themselves, and to take the expert's word for whatever they cannot work out. The precise proportion of those activities in any one instance will depend on the relationship of the complexity of the facts and arguments to the intelligence and motivation of the individual member of the jury. Where this results in the juryman's acceptance of most of the expert's evidence, we have, in effect, 'trial by expert', at least as far as that aspect of the case is concerned. This runs counter to one of the basic principles of English criminal law, that trial in a Crown court shall be by jury. It is the business of the expert to try to explain as much as he reasonably can to the jury, but it is clearly impossible for him to transmit to them his own background of many years' training and practical experience. On their part, the jury must make every effort to understand what the expert is explaining, and in my experience they certainly do try to follow intelligently what is being said to them, but their honest efforts in that direction must be regularly defeated by the sheer complexity of the subject-matter. This topic will be dealt with again in Chapter 6 (The Future).

In the matter of presenting evidence in court, the terms 'evidence-in-chief', 'cross-examination' and 're-examination' are of importance. During the first, the expert states his findings in the case in so far as it concerns him. He would usually be led by counsel in the matter of what he actually did, so he would expect questions of the kind: 'Did you receive a number of tape-recorded speech samples on 5 June 1989?', 'Were you asked to analyse and compare the samples, and to give an opinion as to any possible identification of the speakers?'. However, when the questioning switches to his conclusions, he is no longer led, but instead would be asked, for example: 'Did you come to any conclusion as a result of your examination of the samples?', 'What was that conclusion', and so on. The objective of evidence-in-chief is to allow counsel the opportunity of bringing to the court's notice everything which, in his judgment, will be of use to his case. Usually, all the work the expert has done and the conclusions he has reached are in that category, but it can occur that counsel does not want certain aspects of the witness's role in the case to be heard in court. When that happens, counsel will lead the witness only to those aspects which he does want heard. An example of this, the case of M, is described and discussed in Chapter 5. It should be noted, then, that evidence-in-chief does not necessarily mean that the expert simply stands up and tells the court what opinions he has arrived at and his reasons for doing so. This last point will be discussed in Chapter 6.

Evidence-in-chief is presented as part of either the prosecution's or the defence's case, and the expert is, therefore, on the same side as the relevant counsel. When it comes to cross-examination, however, the converse is true: it is carried out by opposing counsel, and he or she must be expected to attack the expert's evidence. This attack can be either on the expert's evidence as such: his procedures and conclusions, or on his status as an 'expert', or, or course, on both. For an example of a case in which defence counsel attacked the expert's status as such, whilst avoiding mention of his conclusions, see the case of R in Chapter 5. In principle, cross-examination must be based on the witness's evidence-in-chief, but I believe it would be acceptable for new matter to be let in under this heading, presumably in appropriate circumstances. This certainly did not occur in the case of M (Chapter 5), or in any cases in which I have given evidence.

The 'attack' mentioned above may be carried out with varying degrees of vigour and subtlety, and on varying levels of competence, but it is almost always carried out in a courteous manner. In the case of expert witnesses, there may be the added factor of a certain respect being shown by counsel to fellow professionals. In common with other expert witnesses, I have encountered the very occasional opposing counsel who went beyond the bounds of such courtesy in their cross-examination (as in the case of R in Chapter 5). Such counsel, in my opinion, do not bring credit on their profession wherever they are met, but they are, fortunately, untypical and few in number.

'Re-examination' provides counsel with the opportunity of dealing, from his own standpoint, with any matters of importance raised in the cross-examination of his witness. In principle, no new matters may be raised here, but in practice it does occur that new evidence is presented if it can be brought out by following a line of questioning raised by opposing counsel in cross-examination. The case of R in Chapter 5 is a good example of this.

The last heading under which the forensic phonetician might find himself giving evidence is that of 'rebuttal'. This arises when the prosecution has finished its case, and under normal circumstances would not be permitted to present further evidence. However, if the defence have brought evidence of such a nature that the prosecution could not reasonably have expected and made provision for it, the latter could be allowed to introduce evidence in rebuttal of that defence evidence. Everything depends, of course, on the judge's interpretation of 'reasonably'. For example, when defence have introduced a tape-recording without prior warning, prosecution would expect to be allowed to introduce evidence in rebuttal in the form of an expert witness. If, however, prosecution has used recordings of speech samples without calling their own expert to support that presentation, they would probably not be allowed to call such an expert if defence had produced their expert to give an opinion on any aspect of those samples. This kind of situation results in urgent requests for the expert to attend court, and to give evidence if called. In almost all of the cases in which I have been involved, the outcome is an attendance without appearance, because judges, as far as my experience of them goes at least, do not seem to sympathise with arguments from the prosecution concerning the admissibility of rebuttal evidence. If the expert does give evidence, it follows that it is presented under the three headings discussed above.

I have used the term 'identification' on a number of occasions above, but without explanation; it is appropriate now to make such explanation, and to distinguish 'speaker-identification' from 'speaker-recognition', with which it is often confused.

To begin with the latter term: 'speaker-recognition' is what the layman does when he recognises a familiar voice, perhaps over the telephone or in the corridor outside his room, and so on. In the context of everyday life, the phonetician is as much a layman as anybody else as far as this matter is concerned. It is a common experience that we can recognise a known voice from a very short utterance, such as the word 'Hello', or our own name alone 'John', and so on. The processes involved in such an act of recognition are mysterious, in that they seem to be made up of large number of strategies on the part of the 'recogniser', which are not amenable to examination. Obviously, recognition must be based on some aspect or aspects of the speech-signal as it impinges on the ear of the listener, but what those aspects are is not known, and could well vary from person to person, and from case to case. It certainly seems to be true that increasing the length of the sample does not make a great deal of difference to the success of the recognition exercise. Whatever feature the recogniser is fastening upon, he picks it up within the first second or so of the call. If he does not pick it up by then, exposure to more speech rarely makes any difference, unless, of course, verbal clues are mentioned.

'Speaker-identification', on the other hand, is carried out only by the phonetician. This almost invariably involves samples from speakers unknown to him, and his identification is made on the basis of his analysis and comparison of the phonetic characteristics of those samples. The bases of his conclusions are, therefore, overt and testable by other phoneticians, there is nothing in the least mysterious about them. For such phonetic comparisons to be carried out, the samples must be of adequate clarity and substantial content. These latter terms will be discussed at length in Chapter 4, whilst the phonetic features referred to above will be described in the next chapter on phonetics, to which we now turn.

Chapter 2

Phonetics

Most people have heard the word 'phonetics', but if one enquires what they actually think it means, the answers often enough do not have all that much relationship to what phonetics is. In the mind of the layman, 'phonetics' could be associated with something to do with teaching people who cannot speak how to do so, or perhaps it could be something to do with identifying the accent with which a person speaks. There may also be those who think it has something to do with teaching people to speak beautifully and elegantly. There are yet others whose ideas about the subject are mysterious: some years ago a young lady knocked at the door of my office in University College London, and having entered, informed me, without preamble, that she intended to learn about phonetics. I agreed that this would probably be a good idea, and was about to try to find out what kind of course she had in mind when she terminated the interview by saying: 'I won't go into it now, I'll call back later when I've found out something about phonetics'. She disappeared as abruptly as she had arrived, and long before I could utter any useful advice about books, etc. I more or less forgot about her, until, with equal lack of ceremony, she re-appeared a few weeks later. Without mentioning her sources, she announced that she had found out about phonetics, and that she now knew that English had a lot of them, German had some, and Swedish none at all. Since her interests lay in the last language, she now intended to go no further into phonetics, because she obviously did not need 'them'. With that cryptic observation she departed, and I have never seen her again. I therefore have no idea what influence this 'discovery' about phonetics had on her subsequent life and career, and can only hope that she was able to supplant it by better information at some later time. Lay conceptions of what phonetics is, then, seem to range from those in which there is an element of truth,

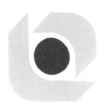

CommsAudit

Chris Mills, I.Eng. F.IEIE
SENIOR CONSULTANT
FORENSIC AUDIO FACILITY

Communications Audit UK Limited.
Network House, Bradfield Close,
Woking, Surrey GU22 7RE, England.
Tel: 0483 750008. (IDD: 44)
Telex: 858802 Remco. Fax: 0483 750166.

such as those relating to accents, via the mistaken, as when the idea of 'beauty' is introduced, to the unfathomable and possibly bizarre, such as the last case.

Obviously, the first task here will have to be to explain the basic principles of phonetics to those who are not adequately versed in them already. I would like to emphasise that this is merely an introduction to or overview of the subject, which I hope will be sufficiently detailed for the layman to make some sense out of the inevitable technical terminology in the coming pages, but not so detailed that he feels burdened with information for which he can find no practical application. In the not entirely impossible event that his curiosity about phonetics is aroused, he will discover that there are many introductory books on the subject, any one of which will provide a vastly more comprehensive cover than is to be found here. I would expect those readers who do know what phonetics is to skip this section, of course.

I think the most important point to remember is that phonetics requires a fundamentally scientific approach to the description of speech, in that it looks on it as a natural object. Phonetics, then, endeavours to treat an act of speech in much the same way as a botanist, for example, would set about describing a leaf, that is, in a totally detached and objective way. Psychologically, this detachment is a great deal easier for the botanist to achieve than for the phonetician. Speech, after all, has been part of our environment since the moment we emerged at birth into a speaking world; there is, in fact, good reason to believe that we are exposed to aspects of speech even before we are born, particularly the rhythmic aspect. As human beings, we are inseparably bound up with speech, in that we treat it as something intimately part of ourselves; we are shaped by speech, and at the same time we generate speech from within ourselves so that we are inclined to believe that it is indivisibly part of our own psyches.

The fundamentally mistaken belief that 'we are what we speak, and we speak what we are' was very nicely illustrated for me some years ago by a neighbour's reaction of bafflement to a situation which a phonetician, or indeed anyone with what I would call the right attitude to speech, would not find in the least problematic. A young girl of the neighbour's acquaintance had started learning Italian from her, and, in order to improve her command of the language and speed up the learning process, the girl arranged to make an extended visit to Italy to stay with an Italian family. On her return some months later she presented herself at my neighbour's house to show off her now confident and fluent Italian. My neighbour was duly impressed, but confessed after the interview that she simply could not understand how the girl could possibly speak Italian 'like a duchess' when her English was 'so common and Cockney'!

Speech, too, is of basic importance in almost every aspect of human activity that one can think of, either speech in its actual spoken form, or in its symbol-equivalent: writing. It is impossible to imagine a society organised without speech. Even in those communities where speech is forbidden for one reason or another, the organisation of each society is based on premises shared by its members, and those premises were inevitably and invariably, at least initially, formulated and acquired through the medium of speech.

Since speech is so basically vital to the organisation and functioning of any form of society known to us, and since we are so intimately involved in speech, it is not in the least surprising, given the character of the human race, that we should be sensitive to its nuances, and that we should evolve prejudices and misconceptions in relation to it, as in the 'We are what we speak . . . ' belief exemplified above. It is a feature of some societies, including and in particular the British, that social class is marked by speech-accent, and that feelings of approval or disapproval with regard to certain accents should be felt on a very fundamental, and often unconscious level. We frequently find that the accent associated with the English establishment is regarded with more approval, i.e. attracts more prestige than do other accents. Despite the profound intuitions to the contrary which are experienced by very many people, the fact that a given accent of speech acquires such prestige is not in the least dependent on any intrinsic virtue of the accent itself, but arises purely as a result of historical circumstances. The prestige accent of English society generally, and it is not in fact restricted to that society, is usually termed 'Received Pronunciation', and is both customarily and conveniently referred to in abbreviation as 'RP'. I shall refer to this accent at any relevant point in the coming pages and without further explanation, as RP.

Phoneticians are, after all, human beings, and as such they are in a somewhat equivocal position: they are, as social animals, subject to the same pressures and prejudices about speech as anyone else, whilst professionally they are required to think and act in an objective manner with regard to that very same object, speech. In their non-professional capacity as ordinary members of society they may very well be heard to express opinions about accents, or an acquaintance's speech habits, such as 'I don't like that accent', or 'I think that's a very soft accent', and so on, i.e. in the context of ordinary social conversation. In their professional personas, however, phoneticians are trained, and successfully trained, of course, to detach from such prejudices, and to treat all forms of speech, even up to and including clinically-deviant speech, not as 'unpleasant' or 'pleasant' etc., etc., but as equally valid, interesting and important targets for description. To sum up, phonetics is a *descriptive* discipline, one therefore in which value judgments are not made. This is a fundamental principle, without which any application or discussion of phonetics, quite simply, cannot be understood. In writing forensic reports or giving evidence in court, I have often used the term: 'Standard Pronunciation' instead of referring explicitly to RP. When I have done this, it has been to circumvent lengthy definitions of the latter term, which is not generally known outside phonetic circles, and certainly not to suggest that it possesses any intrinsic merit or virtue. The privileged status of RP, then, is purely the outcome of a series of accidents in the history of the English language. Naturally, we must make a clear distinction between 'Standard Pronunciation' (which does not exist), and 'Standard Grammar' (which quite obviously does).

Of course, there are many occasions when the material obtained by the *descriptive* approach can and should be applied in a *prescriptive* manner, i.e. actually telling someone how they should pronounce something. Foreign learners of English are a typical example, where some sort of agreed target for their pronunciation must be provided; both in Britain and in many other countries, that target is RP. English-speakers learning a foreign language provide the mirror-image. We must not forget people whose speech has been deviant from birth or which has subsequently become so in some way, e.g. cleft-palate speakers, stroke victims, etc., and, finally, those who wish to change their accents either temporarily, like actors, or permanently, such as speakers who do not like their own native accent. All such people have need of prescribed targets for their pronunciation, though it will not necessarily be RP in all of these cases, of course. If phoneticians are involved in the last type of case, and we would generally prefer not to be, it is only on the understanding that the speaker's decision to change their accent in their own native language is a freedom they enjoy, not a moral and/or civic duty on the part of those speakers. Phoneticians do not make value judgments about accents, but others, such as elocutionists, are in business with that very intent.

In my experience, not all decisions regarding the changing of a speaker's accent in his or her own language have been freely made, however, especially when the subjects concerned are children. In one instance, a left-wing trade union official and his wife decided to send their two daughters to elocution classes. The parents had obviously come to the conclusion that their own accents, if transmitted to their daughters, were not of such a character that would facilitate the entry of the latter to a level of society 'higher', i.e. more prestigious, than their own. The elocutionist was certainly successful in instilling in the girls a form of RP known as 'advanced', typical of the highest levels of professional society; however, unfortunately having lost contact with the family, I have no idea whether the parents' social ambitions, as projected on to their daughters, were ultimately realised or not.

In another instance, a boy from a working-class background won a scholarship from a state school to a school in the private sector. Along with others in the same position, the boy had to devote several hours a week of his school timetable to elocution classes; he was not, of course, consulted on the matter. There sustained efforts were made to change his accent from one appropriate to his family background to one more in keeping with his changed environment. Those efforts were successful in their general intent, but are not recalled with any gratitude by the adult. The elocution classes were timetabled to coincide with Latin classes, and Latin was an obligatory subject for university entrance in those days, so he and those like him were effectively deprived of the opportunity of entering higher education.

Such cases were very common in an earlier generation, and serve as indications of the profound social significance of accent in the British, particularly the English context. Although similar examples could be found today, the earlier, more or less one-way flow of effort towards a prestige accent like RP, is now counterbalanced to some extent by an anti-prestige current. It is a common experience that young people with a social conscience, and from an RP-speaking background, will evince a certain embarrassment at their prestige accent, and take conscious steps to eradicate it, usually in favour of some non-prestigious urban variety.

A further weakening influence on the prestige of RP in its traditional function of securing preferential treatment for its speakers when they seek entry to high-status employment, is to be found in any of the modern, highly-technologised industries. Here the only requirements of the employee are consistent and successful performance, together with the confident manipulation of high technology; little interest seems to be accorded the speaker's accent. If the evidence of their speech as heard in televised interviews at times of financial crisis is to be believed, it is certainly true to say that one does not have to speak RP to be a 'whizz kid' in the City!

It will be clear, I hope, that it is not the business of phoneticians to volunteer instructions as to how people should pronounce their own languages. When Daniel Jones founded the world's first university phonetics department in 1907 at University College London, he provoked the outrage of George Bernard Shaw by establishing it in strict accordance with the descriptive principle. The latter had hoped for an institution from which would emanate precepts for the native speaker of English as to how English should be pronounced, just as the Académie Française does for French speakers of French. Shaw seemed to believe that the English were particularly slovenly and inept in pronouncing their own language, and therefore needed rather more than usual pressure and advice in that direction. Jones's failure to subscribe to that Shavian misconception gave rise to a disagreement which was to survive both of them beyond the grave.

Readers will be greatly helped in their understanding of the nature of speech if they are able to appreciate that speech is multi-dimensional: it exists simultaneously in many different aspects and on many levels. One of the most important of these levels of speech is that of speech production, and we should not be surprised to discover that this has many aspects: the internal, mental processes of generating speech, the articulatory movements made by the organs of speech, such as the lips and tongue (the organs of speech, from the lips and nostrils externally to the larynx internally, are known collectively as 'the vocal tract'); the external appearance of the person when speaking, as for example when the lips can be seen to be rounded; the sounds the listener hears, and the physical disturbances in the air which the speech-act produces. We could, perhaps, add the ways in which the listener hears the sounds. Of all of these aspects, only those which can be directly observed form the subject-matter for phonetics:

1. The movements of the organs of speech on the part of the speaker.
2. The sounds which are produced.

These features are classified and measured in a variety of ways.

When the disturbances in the external air are measured by electronic devices this is referred to as acoustic phonetics; there is a separate chapter devoted to this aspect of speech-analysis (Chapter 3 - Acoustic Phonetics), in which its role in forensic phonetics is also discussed and evaluated. Otherwise sounds are classified according to their articulatory and/or auditory characteristics, i.e. which organs of speech are used in their production, and what they sound like. However, before any sound can be produced in the vocal tract, one fundamental requirement must be satisfied: there must be a movement of air within the tract which is then modified in various ways. In the vast majority of speech sounds in any language this movement is of air set in motion by the lungs, and in an outward direction; it is in consequence known as the egressive pulmonic (lung) airstream. Some speech sounds are produced with other airstreams, for example the click sounds used in some southern African languages are made on an airstream initiated in the mouth (oral cavity), and ingressively, i.e. with air going in. The use of air going into the lungs - ingressive pulmonic - is extremely rare in speech. The first classification of speech sounds, then, must be in terms of the airstream used. In practice this is not usually mentioned, though, because one can reasonably assume that speech sounds *are* produced on an egressive pulmonic airstream unless it is specifically stated to the contrary.

The first organ of speech encountered by the air from the lungs is the larynx. This is a highly complex organ, with commensurately complex functions which can only be dealt with very simply here: it is responsible for the basic 'buzz' of the voice, and also for the features of pitch and loudness. The buzz referred to is known as 'voice', and this itself is far from simple, since it may encompass different 'voice-qualities', such as 'falsetto', and the relatively self-explanatory 'creaky' and 'breathy' voice. In the description of speech sounds, it is a matter of vital importance to discover whether voice is present or not, whether, in other words, those sounds are 'voiced' or 'voiceless'. Even this last statement is an over-simplification, but a necessary one for reasons of brevity. As we shall see below, certain kinds of sounds can more or less be assumed to be voiced, whereas others are unpredictable in terms of the voice feature – it could equally well be present or absent.

The features of speech can helpfully be divided into two broad categories: 'segmental' and 'supra-segmental'. Let us begin with a description of the segmental category, which consists, basically, of what the layman would feel he understands: vowels and consonants. Although there are a number of intermediate, borderline cases where the boundary is not as obvious as the layman would suppose, for the most part the terms 'vowel' and 'consonant' mean more or less what the layman thinks they mean. It would not be helpful for the reader who is not specially interested in the subject to have rehearsed here the lengthy arguments concerning the precise definitions of these terms to be found in many phonetics textbooks. Furthermore, such definitions could not, for example, conceivably constitute the topic of any dispute in the forensic area.

By far the most widespread and accepted approach to the description of vowel sounds is the one based on the concept of 'auditory reference qualities', or *Cardinal Vowels*. These are, basically, a set of vowel qualities established, fixed and maintained *by ear*. The qualities were devised by Daniel Jones in the first instance (see Figures 2.1 and 2.2), although they have subsequently required additions and other changes, in order to maintain them in their practical role of serving as descriptive reference points for phoneticians to use in describing the vowels of any form of human speech. A glance at the just-revised chart of the International Phonetic Association will make clear the present character of the symbols and descriptive terms which phoneticians have at their disposal for describing vowels. Any trained phonetician, therefore, would expect his verbal or symbol-based description of a given vowel sound to be correctly interpreted by another phonetician, i.e. he should be able to

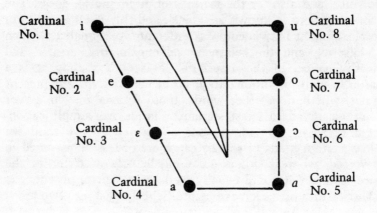

Figure 2.1 Conventionalized diagram illustrating the tongue positions
of the cardinal vowels

reproduce the 'same' sound as the describer had in mind. In fact,
this could only be the same sound with respect to the features
of speech included in the descriptive framework - in keeping
with the rest of humanity, phoneticians come in a wide variety
of shapes and sizes, and for this reason it will, I hope, be obvious
that no two of them will sound alike in every possible respect,
but they will nevertheless be able to select certain features of
speech and reproduce those in the manner described above. As
the reader will see on the chart, current terminology relates to
the notional position of the tongue in terms of its relative
height in the mouth (close/open, for example), and its relative
frontness or backness (front/back, etc.). I have use the word
'notional' advisedly, since the relationship between the shape
and position of the tongue and the auditory quality of the vowel
is not absolute, but subject to variation in a number of
parameters - within the speech of the same person through
time, and/or from one speaker to another, for example. This
variation might well prove an interesting topic for basic
research, but such research cannot, by its very nature, find a
place in the forensic field, where the demands are of such an
immediate character. It must logically be the case that the
auditory quality of the vowel is the only one which is relevant
in the day-to-day practical applications of phonetics, and

forensics is a major example of such applications. The attentive reader will have noticed that there is no explicit dimension of lip-shape on the chart. This aspect of description is intrinsic to the choice of symbol – some symbols are more or less arbitrarily designated to relate to rounded vowels, whilst others are used to denote vowels produced either with spread lips or with a neutral lip-shape.

Readers will also observe that the section on 'diacritics' includes many, perhaps to them odd-looking signs. Without burdening them with lengthy explanations as to the precise functions of these diacritics, I would ask them to note that they enable phoneticians to render vowel sounds in an even more accurate way than simply using vowel symbols would, because, by judiciously adding them to those symbols, they are able to reach the more subtle nuances of quality which would otherwise elude description. Phoneticians tend to regard the descriptive resources offered by the unmodified Cardinal Vowel symbols as relatively crude and inadequate.

Consonants are customarily described on a rather different basis from that of vowel description. This difference derives from a difference between vowels and consonants in their fundamental character: vowels are generally produced without firm contact of any part of the tongue with any area of the fixed parts of the mouth, whereas consonants do tend to have some kind of contact. (As I mentioned a little earlier, this is not a rigid categorisation – there are many intermediate cases – but the generality is sufficiently valid for us to be able to formulate different descriptive frameworks for vowels and consonants.) Referring back to the question of whether sounds are usually voiced or voiceless: it will probably be clear now that vowels typically have no noise component (because they involve no contact) and must, if they are to be audible, be produced with voicing. Consonants, on the other hand, typically do have a noise component (because they usually require some degree of contact), and consequently can be clearly heard whether they are accompanied by voice or not.

One very important and far-reaching result of this difference is that vowels need to be described, principally, in what is effectively an auditory manner, despite the pseudo-articulatory labels such as 'close', 'front', etc. It is, I think, obvious that one could not respond in any meaningful way to an instruction of the sort: 'Raise your tongue until the back is halfway between the

CONSONANTS

	Bilabial	Labiodental	Dental	Alveolar	Postalveolar	Retroflex	Palatal	V
Plosive	p b			t d		ʈ ɖ	c ɟ	k
Nasal	m	ɱ		n		ɳ	ɲ	
Trill	ʙ			r				
Tap or Flap				ɾ		ɽ		
Fricative	ɸ β	f v	θ ð	s z	ʃ ʒ	ʂ ʐ	ç ʝ	x
Lateral fricative				ɬ ɮ				
Approximant		ʋ		ɹ		ɻ	j	
Lateral approximant				l		ɭ	ʎ	
Ejective stop	p'			t'		ʈ'	c'	k'
Implosive	ɓ ɓ			ƭ ɗ			ƈ ʄ	ƙ

Where symbols appear in pairs, the one to the right represents a voiced consonant. Shaded areas den

DIACRITICS

̥	Voiceless	n̥ d̥	̹	More rounded	ɔ̹	ʷ	Labialized	tʷdʷ	̃	Nasa
̌	Voiced	s̬ t̬	̜	Less rounded	ɔ̜	ʲ	Palatalized	tʲdʲ	ⁿ	Nasa
ʰ	Aspirated	tʰ dʰ	̟	Advanced	u̟	ˠ	Velarized	tˠdˠ	ˡ	Later
̈	Breathy voiced	b̤ a̤	̠	Retracted	i̠	ˤ	Pharyngealized	tˤ dˤ	˥	No au
̰	Creaky voiced	b̰ a̰	̈	Centralized	ë	~	Velarized or pharyngealized		
̼	Linguolabial	t̼ d̼	̽	Mid centralized	ě	̝	Raised	e̝ ɹ̝	
̪	Dental	t̪ d̪	̘	Advanced Tongue root	e̘		(ɹ̝ = voiced alveolar fricative)		
̺	Apical	t̺ d̺	̙	Retracted Tongue Root	e̙	̞	Lowered	e̞ β̞	
̻	Laminal	t̻ d̻	˞	Rhoticity	ə˞		(β̞ = voiced bilabial approxim		
						̩	Syllabic	ɬ̩	̯	Non-

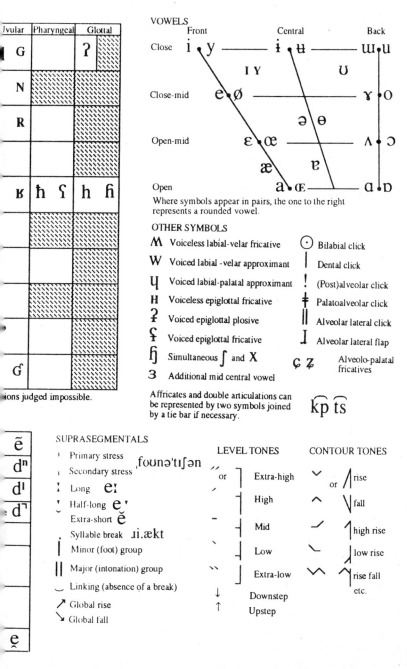

Figure 2.2 The international phonetic alphabet (revised to 1989)

tongue's lowest position and the roof of the mouth.' This is, in fact, what one would have to do to produce a specific vowel quality; clearly, an auditorily-based approach is more likely to achieve success, i.e. one in which straightforward imitation is underpinned by knowledge of the Cardinal Vowel theory and practice. With the exception of lip-shape and one or two other cases, articulatorily-based instructions concerning the performance of designated vowel qualities are uninterpretable.

Looked at from another point of view, if a speaker introspects, and uses their kinaesthetic sense to attempt to discover what is going on in articulatory terms in their mouths when they produce a given sound, they are not likely to come up with anything very positive when they try the experiment with vowels. They will be able to feel little of what is happening, with the exception of the shape of the lips and a few extreme vowel postures. This is far from being the case with consonantal articulations, though, and our system of classifying consonants is, therefore, based principally on the effectiveness of introspection. This technique is employed in Catford's challenging book, and will not be further developed here. It will suffice to say that we are naturally more easily aware of the activities of the tip and blade of the tongue, and the lips than we are of those areas of the vocal tract which lie further back. It follows from this that the 'place of articulation' labels which phoneticians conventionally use for describing consonants will be more immediately intelligible to the layman when they relate to sounds produced using both lips: 'bilabial'; bottom lip and top teeth: 'labio-dental'; tongue tip/blade and alveolar ridge: 'alveolar', etc. When the articulators are further back, e.g. front of the tongue and the hard palate: 'palatal'; back of the tongue and the soft palate: 'velar'; back of the tongue and the uvula: 'uvular', and so on, the labels are less transparent in their meanings.

It was mentioned above that speech exists on many levels, and it is necessary, before going any further, for us to enlarge on one of the implications of that statement. A simple example will help us get to the point in the most direct way. If we consider the 'l' sounds in words like 'let' and 'tell' in RP or any accent roughly approaching RP, it is interesting to note the layman's response to the question: 'Does the same sound occur at the beginning of the first word as at the end of the second word?' His first reaction is invariably to say 'Yes'. He is quite right in this reaction, of course, but if we then ask him to listen very carefully to the actual *sounds* in each case, he usually perceives some difference between them. Naturally, he is not in a position to describe that difference in phonetic terms, but the fact remains that he has noticed a real difference. If his first reaction was right, i.e. that the sounds are the same, and if his second conclusion is also right, i.e. that they are different, then he is clearly making contradictory statements. In fact, the two contradictory statements about 'sameness' here are not really mutually exclusive, because they are made about two different levels in the analysis of speech. The second judgment relates to the precise observation of the sounds *per se* in the phonetic sense that we have been talking about in the preceding pages, and the observation that the sounds are phonetically different is, therefore, correct on that level. The first reaction was also correct, as we will no doubt feel in an intuitive way, but this time the sameness is of a rather more abstract kind. This level is the subject of a good deal of controversy, none of which, fortunately, is of relevance in an introductory work of this nature. The most important point to remember is that many linguists, including, of course, phoneticians, accept the two levels of which we are speaking as useful, if not necessarily essential components of their analyses of speech. The more abstract level can be referred to as the 'phonemic' level, and the units which constitute this level are usually termed 'phonemes'. Returning to our earlier example: the words 'let' and 'tell' have the same 'l' phoneme, customarily enclosed in slanting brackets: /l/, but each occurrence of that phoneme is phonetically different. Such phonetically different segments, when spoken of in relation to phonemes, are known as 'variants', 'allophones' or 'realisations' of that phoneme, and the relevant symbols would be enclosed in [ ] (there is no need for the reader to be occupied with the symbols).

The system of phonemes for all RP speakers is more or less the same, but regional speakers of RP, such as those from London, will often have realisations which show their regional origins. For example, RP speakers are likely to have a 'pure vowel' (or 'monophthong' - a steady quality throughout the syllable) in words like: 'bee', whereas London speakers could be heard to use a 'diphthong' (two vowel qualities in the same syllable). Other accents could well be different from RP in their phonemic systems and/or in their phonetic features. Organisation of the raw material of speech - the highly variable phonetic events described in the Introduction – into a phonemic system is one of the principle areas in which interpretation by the analyser plays a vital part.

Turning to supra-segmental characteristics; these are, as the name suggests, features which characteristically extend over more than one segment. Pitch is the most important of those features, and it, too, has to be considered from a number of points of view.

Pitch relates to the musical note which is inevitably present when the larynx produces voice, and one way in which this musical characteristic can be exploited in describing speech is to refer to its average pitch. This can be measured instrumentally, or arrived at by the auditory process. In the latter case the judgment can either be stated in absolute terms, in relation to some conventional musical scale, for example, or relativistically, comparing an utterance with some notional average pitch, and/or comparing the average pitch of one utterance with that of another. In the forensic context, I do not think that average pitch by itself is a very strong indexical feature, i.e. it does not constitute a reliable indicator of an individual speaker. The first case in Chapter 5 is such an instance, where a clear difference of average pitch between two long speech samples was not indicative of two different speakers, but was to be explained in terms of the different mental states of the same speaker. In the case quoted the pitch judgments were performed auditorily, and were, therefore, fairly approximate. Instrumental measurements, on the other hand, are very much more accurate, and are specifiable in numerical terms, as is explained in Chapter 3. However, I would not be happy to conclude from this that an instrumentally-measured pitch difference between two speech samples would be any more reliable, in itself, as an indicator that those samples were probably spoken by two different people than one which was auditorily-based. The greater the pitch discrepancy, of course, the more inclined I would be to consider it of potential significance, but the principle for me remains: no matter how great the pitch differences, and no matter how they were measured, I would always hope for further negative indications. These would be most convincing if they were of a segmental character.

The other major aspect of pitch is in its role in intonation. This term refers to the pitch variations within an utterance, its tune, in other words. Intonation, too, can be analysed either

instrumentally, or in purely musical terms by auditory reference
to the notes of a musical scale.

Otherwise, description could be phrased in either a non-
systemic or a systemic way. Both of these methods are auditory.
The first takes the form of impressionistic and relativistic dots
and dashes, resembling tadpoles as much as anything else, and
representing the speaker's pitch levels and/or pitch movements.
These tadpoles are usually located between two parallel lines
notionally representative of the speaker's upper and lower pitch
limits. There are other graphic ways in which the same result
could be achieved, but whichever variant is chosen, notation of
this kind is very powerful because it can get to the finest
nuances of the intonation tune.

Not all analyses are based on the premise that every pitch
event needs to be noted explicitly, however. A systemic
analysis, for example, starts from the assumption that general-
isations can be made about pitch features, such that many
details of pitch can be subsumed under broader headings. The
requirements of a systemic analysis are very different from a
non-systemic analysis. In the latter, as described above, it is
extremely important to note every pitch detail, along with
features relating to the rhythmic structure which will be
explained below. In the case of a systemic analysis, however, a
more abstract approach is necessary. Pitch features which would
be noted separately in a non-systemic analysis, can be subsumed
in the same systemic category so long as two conditions are
met: there should be a basic similarity amongst the pitch details
included in that category, and the reactions of native speakers
to the occurrence in speech of any of those different pitch
features must be demonstrably, or at least arguably, the same.
Let us consider a very simple example: it is very common in RP
to hear a tune which falls and then rises within a single-syllable
word such as 'Yes'. If we examine the detailed pitch characteristics of a number of such occurrences, we will find that the
same speaker produces the generalised fall-rise in many different
ways: starting and/or ending higher or lower; widening or
narrowing the overall pitch range; changing the voice-quality on
the lowest pitch level, and so on. We must first discover
whether the listener does in fact perceive and react to these
different events in the same way. In this case we will
consistently get the same response to our enquiry: 'the speaker
is signalling grudging and/or partial agreement'. If the roles are

reversed, and the above speaker becomes the listener, he will accept as 'the same', tunes from another speaker which are markedly different from his own. Given such confirmation of our hypothesis, we are justified in considering all the pitch variations just described as realisations of a single abstract systemic unit, which is customarily termed 'the fall-rise'. Had the listener experienced different reactions to any of those variations, for example, had he felt that a different signal was intended by the speaker when he started the tune on a lower pitch than he ended it on, then that would have justified the setting-up of two abstract systemic units, and so on. The principle is that one establishes as many such units as seems functionally necessary to the analyser.

It might, perhaps, be appropriate at this point to remind the reader that computers are, at the present time, unable to assist in the cerebral operation of establishing an abstract system from a mass of complex pitch data.

Such systemic units are usually known as 'nuclear tones'. In my department we generally operate with seven nuclear tones, but whatever the number and nature of the tones in any other analysis, they have other functions than signalling attitudes of the kind described above. The most important of these functions is to show the location(s) in an utterance of what we call 'focus'. Without entering into lengthy discussions of what is both a complex and a fascinating subject, I would here offer what must be an over-simplified definition of focus, as 'the highlighting within an utterance of words or topics which the speaker wishes to draw to the listener's attention'. Where such highlighting occurs, the selected item bears a nuclear tone, and is considered to be the site of the 'nucleus'. Some examples will, I hope, make this clear. If we take the sentence: 'Jack's bought a new car', we can locate the nuclear tone, and therefore the nucleus, anywhere that we wish in order to signal our selected focus:

1. 'Jack's bought a new *car*.' This has either broad focus, indicating a general interest in all the items in the sentence, or a narrow focus on 'car', possibly contrasting it with 'bicycle' which a listener could be assuming.
2. 'Jack's bought a *new* car.' Here focus is narrow, contrasting 'new' with the expected 'second-hand'.

From these examples it will be obvious to the reader that,

indeed, any word can be the site of the nucleus, and consequently of focus – even 'a', which could possibly imply that the speaker did not know the make of car, or, perhaps, correcting an earlier statement or assumption to the effect that Jack had bought several new cars. It is important to remember that the placement of focus is never arbitrary or random; all utterances fit into a specific context of communication, and the speaker selects what is relevant to that context. Location of nucleus is one of the variables checked by the phonetician when describing natural speech, and any unusual feature(s) would be noted.

The parallels between system of intonation and system of segmental units (phonemes) will not, I hope, escape the reader.

The final supra-segmental feature to be described is that of the rhythmic aspect of speech, which, in RP, can be expressed in terms of the contrast between 'strong' and 'weak' syllables. Every utterance in RP has at least one strong syllable. If that utterance is a monosyllable, then, self-evidently, that single syllable must be strong, e.g. 'man'. However, if the utterance has two syllables, it is possible for one of those syllables to be strong and the other weak, as in 'manner', where the first syllable is strong and the second weak. If we look at a three-syllable utterance like 'manager' we can perceive that its rhythmic structure is strong + weak + weak. There are obviously very many possible permutations; without my listing every conceivable combination it might be interesting for the reader to note that the order and co-occurrence of strong/weak syllables is fairly free. This means that weak can precede strong, as in the verb 'diffuse', as contrasted with a different verb 'defuse', which, for almost all RP speakers except television news readers, has two strong syllables. It is important to remember at this point that intonation both interrelates with and functions independently of rhythm; in the case of 'defuse', for example, the second syllable will be rendered more prominent, but not stronger than the first by the presence of an intonation nucleus on the second syllable. (An intonation nucleus must be located on a strong syllable, but strong syllables may occur in the absence of a nucleus, as in the first syllable of 'defuse'.) So far, utterances have been assumed to consist of single words, but that is, of course, far from being the case in real life. However the utterance is made up, whether it be of monosyllables, longer words, or any combination of them, the rhythmic structure of those utterances can be deemed to be expressible in the same terms. For example, the following two utterances would be considered to have the same rhythmic structure:

*Sell*afield v. *Sell* a field

where the second utterance would fit into a conversation of the sort:

'I want to raise some quick money from my farm. Should I rent or sell a field?'
'Sell a field.'

The two utterances under discussion do not, however, have the same grammatical structure, and because of this, the perceptive reader will probably find that they do not actually sound exactly the same. A further investigation into these differences and their causes would certainly prove fascinating, but would take us far beyond the scope of this book.

In an utterance it is possible to find that every word carries a rhythmic beat. For example, it would be perfectly normal in the following sentence to have the structure:

'*Jill ran quickly from her hou*se',

where the stressed syllables are italicised. This would probably be perceived as rather an emphatic way of speaking, though, and a more usual structure would perhaps be:

'*Jill* ran *quick*ly from her *house*'.

Here we have actually removed, or deleted, three of the original six rhythmic beats. If we now concentrate on the words 'ran', 'from' and 'her' in each sentence, we will almost certainly notice that the words last longer in the first example than in the second. This difference is the result of a feature characteristic of RP and most other accents of English, whereby the duration of a syllable depends on its location in the rhythmic structure: if it carries a beat it lasts longer, but if that beat is deleted, the syllable is made shorter. One consequence of this is that in English we feel that the length of an utterance depends on the number of rhythmic beats, not the number of syllables; for us, therefore, the first sentence is twice as long as the second. In French, for example, it would be the other way round, so that both sentences would have the same length, háving the same number of syllables. For this reason, English is usually referred to as a 'stress-timed' language, whereas French is a 'syllable-timed' language.

A further consequence of the deletion of rhythmic beats on 'from' and 'her' is that different vowel qualities are heard, as well as, possibly, other changes such as the dropping of /h/ in 'her'. It will be noted that no such changes take place on 'ran', which is subject only to the reduction in duration. English words thus divide into two broad categories: those like 'ran', i.e. verbs, nouns, adjectives and adverbs, which do not permit reduction of vowel qualities, etc., and the remaining group like 'from' and 'her', i.e. prepositions, pronouns, etc., which do.

Many foreign speakers of English fail to make the kind of vowel reduction described above. In the English of many native speakers of West African languages, as well as in the speech of many West Indians, one can observe both that omission and the presence of syllable timing.

This brings us to the last item in the list of supra-segmental features: loudness. Variations in loudness are achieved in the larynx by opening the vocal folds more or less widely when they are vibrating (producing, respectively, louder and quieter speech), and for whatever section of the utterance the speaker chooses. Greater loudness could coincide with a whole sentence, therefore, or be associated with a single syllable. In the latter case it could be considered to account, if only in part, for the difference between a strong syllable and a weak one.

We have now reached the end of our brief and superficial overview of the subject of phonetics. I should perhaps remind the reader that all the topics described in the immediately preceding pages fall potentially into the forensic area of activity. I have often been asked whether phonetic comparisons are like fingerprint matching, i.e. based on a 'points of comparison' system which is expressed numerically. The reader will now, I hope, be in a position to appreciate why such a one-dimensional scale would be quite inappropriate for phonetic comparison.

Chapter 3

Acoustic Phonetics

Introduction

It is becoming increasingly common to find tape-recordings submitted as evidence in English criminal trials. Although it is by no means a rare occurrence for the defence to submit such evidence, in the vast majority of trials it is the prosecution that relies upon recordings in presenting its case.

Evidential recordings produced by the prosecution usually involve a speaker who is claimed to be the defendant either committing a crime by means of voice (for example, making an indecent telephone call or issuing an illegal threat), or saying something that implicates him in a criminal act (for instance, making a confession).

Tape-recorded evidence of this type is often challenged by the defence. Typically, the defence challenge takes one or more of the following three forms:

1. It may be claimed that the voice in the recording is not that of the defendant.
2. It may be claimed that the prosecution's interpretation of the recorded speech is erroneous, that is, that the person responsible for making a written transcript of the recording has misheard or misrepresented what was said.
3. It may be claimed that the recording has been edited or otherwise tampered with.

The services of forensic phoneticians are called upon in order to ascertain the validity of all three types of challenge, and in this chapter I shall be concerned to describe some of the methods and tests that I have used to this end. Particular attention will be given to the role of instrumental analyses in this respect.

Speaker identification

In previous chapters of this book, attention has focused upon the uses of auditory phonetic analysis in arriving at an opinion on whether two or more samples of speech were produced by the same person. For reasons explained later in this chapter, my own view is that an auditory phonetic analysis is absolutely essential to the speaker identification task. However, it is also my contention that the task should not *only* include an auditory analysis. There are at least two good reasons for believing that auditory phonetic analyses coupled with instrumental, or acoustic, tests provides the best way forward for the expert witness involved in this area.

The first and most general reason is that a conclusion which is based upon results deriving from two different kinds of examination is stronger than a conclusion based wholly upon the results of one. One might draw an analogy here with another area of forensic science: that of the pathologist attempting to provide an estimation of the time of death from a body.

There are various methods available for making such an assessment. For instance, the pathologist might take the temperature of the corpse, and drawing upon his knowledge of mass tissue cooling rates after death, within given external atmospheric temperatures, attempt an assessment by this method. If, however, the time of the deceased person's last meal were known, it might also be possible to assess the death time from an examination of the state of the digestion of the stomach's contents. Further, if insect larvae were found on the body, then the time could be estimated from an investigation of their state of development.

Obviously, an opinion based upon two of these factors would be better than an opinion formed on the basis of just one. An opinion which took account of all three would be more reliable still.

Similarly, with speech comparisons, an opinion founded upon auditory *and* acoustic examinations of the samples must be seen as stronger and more dependable than one based solely upon auditory investigations.

The second reason for undertaking acoustic as well as auditory analyses concerns the fact that there are aspects of speech we now know to be relevant to the identification task which one can only examine or measure instrumentally. Long-term pitch average, as discussed below, is an example of this. If one is not simply to ignore these factors, acoustic tests must be carried out.

Acoustic examinations

What is meant by the terms 'acoustic' or 'instrumental' examinations?

Briefly stated, acoustic phonetics is the branch of phonetic study which is concerned with the analysis of speech as a set of vibration patterns, or sound waves. A good introduction to the concepts associated with this area is provided in Fry (1979). My approach here will be to provide practical illustrations of some of the main tests undertaken, introducing only such information as is necessary for an understanding of what is involved.

Acoustic examinations of speech samples are carried out upon each of the areas of speech examined auditorily. That is, as part of the speaker identification procedure, I would normally undertake acoustic examinations of pitch, of segmental features (vowels and consonants), and, where practicable, of certain aspects of voice quality.

Pitch

When we speak, air is exhaled from the body. On its route from the lungs to the outside world the air passes through the larynx, a box-like structure composed of cartilage, a hard but pliable tissue. The function of the larynx is to protect two thick strips of muscle known as the 'vocal cords'.

As was explained in Chapter 2, consonant sounds may be divided into two groups: voiced and voiceless. With voiced consonants – and indeed all vowels – the vocal cords vibrate rapidly as the lung air passes between them on its way through the larynx. The vibratory action of the vocal cords is transferred to the air itself. When the airwave impinges upon the ear of the listener it is vibrating at a basic rate which corresponds to the rate of vocal cord vibration. The perceptual effect created by this vibration is known as 'pitch'. The faster the rate of vibration, the higher pitched we hear the voice to be. Thus, women, who

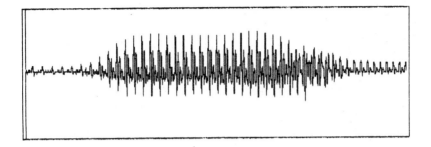

Figure 3.1 Waveform of one speaker's pronunciation of the word
'ZOOM'

for physiological reasons, have a faster rate of vocal cord vibration than men, are heard as having higher voices than men.

Figure 3.1 is of a graph made by computer program of the
waveform of one speaker's pronunciation of the word ZOOM
(voiced throughout). The horizontal axis of the graph represents
time, and the vertical dimension reflects amplitude. Each of the
major vertical striations corresponds to one vibration of the
vocal cords.

Pitch is measured instrumentally in terms of the number of
vibrations that occur per second. The unit of measurement used
here is known as 'CPS' (cycles per second), or, more commonly,
'Hz' (an abbreviation for 'Hertz').

There is a good deal of pitch variation, both across the population and within the speech of any individual. However, research
undertaken by Dr Hermann Künzel of the Speaker Identification
Department of the Bundeskriminalamt (Federal Police) in West
Germany suggests that each speaker has a relatively stable
average pitch height which can be calculated with a good degree
of reliability, providing one makes the calculation on the basis
of around two minutes or more of speech, and is careful to
exclude from the analysis any sections which show a high
degree of emotion.

Individual pitch averages can be calculated using a variety of
different instrumental methods. The most commonly used one
involves re-recording the speech digitally within a computer
system, and having the calculation made by a computer
program designed for this purpose.

Programs for pitch extraction can provide their result in the

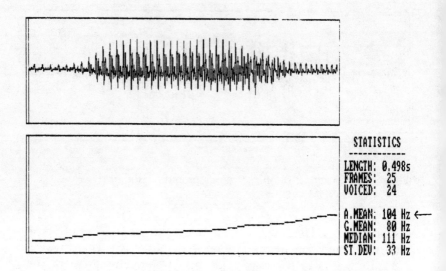

Figure 3.2 Pitch trace and pitch average calculation for word 'ZOOM'

form of a number and/or a graphic illustration on the computer screen of the varying pitch contour of the speech above a representation of its waveform. Figure 3.2 again shows the rendering of the word ZOOM represented in Figure 3.1.

Here the average (mean) pitch of the speech appears as the figure of 104 Hz marked by an arrow at the right-hand side of the bottom window. The bottom window shows the direction of pitch movement over the word. One can see that the pitch rises, first quite steeply, then more shallowly, and finally more steeply again, over the duration of the word.

A central advantage of this type of program is that it is capable of handling extended stretches of speech. Figure 3.3 below shows a fundamental frequency trace and the calculated average pitch for around 19 seconds of speech (100 Hz).

In undertaking identification tasks, it is in my view important that, wherever possible, two minutes of speech from both the known and the disputed samples are analysed in this way, and the average fundamental frequencies compared. In many cases in which I have been involved, where there has been independent evidence that the two samples were produced by the same person, the average pitch has matched to within 5 Hz (a little less than one semi-tone).

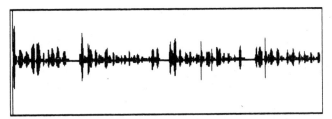

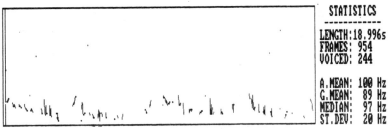

STATISTICS

LENGTH:18.996s
FRAMES: 954
VOICED: 244

A.MEAN: 100 Hz
G.MEAN: 89 Hz
MEDIAN: 97 Hz
ST.DEV: 20 Hz

Figure 3.3 Pitch trace and pitch average calculation for 19 seconds of speech

If the average pitch between the two samples is widely different, then this is taken as a counter-indication to the proposition that they have been produced by the same person, unless, of course, the samples match closely in other respects, and factors are present (e.g. illness, excitement, stress) which would explain the pitch difference.

The significance one can attach to the finding that two samples are of similar average pitch is to an extent dependent upon what that average is. Population statistics have been compiled on the percentages of men and women in given age bands who share particular pitch averages. So, for example, we know that in the population of males aged between twenty and sixty years an average pitch of 115-118 Hz is very common. The finding that a disputed speech sample and a known sample from a male aged thirty years both fell within this range, then, would not, in itself, be treated as greatly significant. However, if the disputed and known samples showed pitch averages of, respectively, 174 Hz and 170 Hz - as recently happened in a case in which I acted - then much greater importance would be attached to the match, as research indicates this pitch average is found in less than 1.0% of the male population aged 20-60.

48   *Forensic Phonetics*

In addition to individuals varying in their average pitch, they also vary in terms of the *pitch range* they exploit. Whilst the speech of some people is rather monotonous and mainly constrained within a narrow pitch band, that of others shows frequent and wide variation. The statistical measure of this variation is known as 'standard deviation from the mean'. If there is frequent oscillation between very different pitch values, the standard deviation will be represented as a greater figure than if there is not.

Certain computer programs for pitch analysis will make automatic calculations of standard deviation from the mean. In Figure 3.3, this figure (20 Hz) has been entered at the foot of the column of figures to the right of the bottom window.

I am presently engaged in research to establish how consistent individuals are in terms of this aspect of pitch. Initial indications are that standard deviation remains reasonably stable within the speech of individuals and varies quite widely across speakers.

The third aspect of pitch measured instrumentally in speaker identification cases is *intonation*. Speakers who share a similar average pitch may vary in the terms of the nuclear tones they habitually choose.

Tone choice is of particular significance where the patterns found are aberrant or idiosyncratic. In one case which involved comparing a known sample of voice from a suspect with that of a malicious telephone caller to the fire service, both samples showed extended series of tone units containing level or slightly rising tonics. Many speakers do make use of this intonation pattern, but they do so when listing events or items ('tea, coffee, sugar . . .'). In this case no listing was involved. Pitch traces produced by computer program, including those in Figures 3.4 and 3.5, were used to establish the degree of similarity between the samples in terms of this idiosyncratic feature and to provide the court with a graphic record of it.

Segmental features

In my own practice, acoustic examinations of vowels and consonants are carried out selectively. If, on the basis of an auditory examination of the samples, I consider that the pronunciation of certain vowels or consonants may serve as an

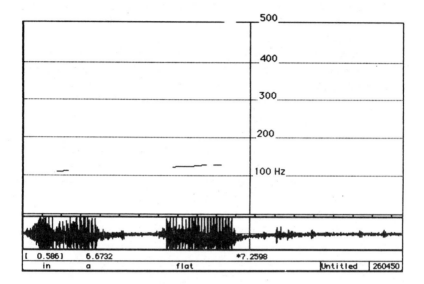

Figure 3.4 Pitch trace showing use of level tone by malicious caller

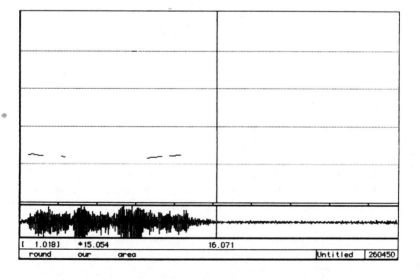

Figure 3.5 Pitch trace showing use of level tone by suspect

individual distinguishing feature or as evidence that different speakers were involved, then I examine instances of those sounds instrumentally.

There are two main aspects of vowels and consonants which can be measured by acoustic analysis: their timings and their frequency structure.

Measurements of timings

A recent case involving charges of theft and indecent telephone calls provides an interesting illustration of how the timing of speech segments may be significant in speaker identifications.

The case involved a young man who had broken into the house of a women, stolen items of underwear, and subsequently telephoned her to discuss them.

The known sample of voice, taken from a recording of a police interview with the suspect, showed evidence of stammering. Stammering is sub-divided into three types: repetition, block, and prolongation. Repetition refers to the tendency, more often found in children than in adults, to recycle or repeat either individual consonants or syllables. Block and prolongation refer to slightly different problems concerning the timing of consonants.

Block is the tendency to arrest the development of certain consonants, in particular plosives. So, for example, with a /d/, the tongue may be held in contact with the alveolar ridge for a longer than normal time, there being some neuro-motor impediment to its release (the 'block'). Prolongation is most often associated with fricatives, and refers to the tendency to sustain them beyond their normal duration.

Evidence of both block and prolongation was discovered from an auditory examination of the samples.

Parts of both samples were re-recorded within a computer system and consonants exhibiting block and prolongation were identified. A computer program was run producing *sound spectrograms* of the relevant sections of speech. Spectrograms are graphs which show both the timings of particular sounds and their frequency components. The spectrographic records showed that the timing of the consonants subject to block and sustension was very similar across the known and disputed samples. For example, /t/ and /d/ were most subject to block where they occurred in word-final position. The hold phase of blocked /t/ and /d/ had a minimum duration of just over 0.2 seconds (around the time most English speakers take to articulate a stressed syllable) and a maximum of 1.5 seconds, the average being 0.4 in both samples.

/s/, and /f/ were most prominent among the consonants that showed prolongation, the average length being closely matched, again at around 0.4 seconds across the known and disputed samples.

The incidence of stammering in general in the adult male population is calculated at around 1.0% (Enderby and Phillip, 1986). No figures are available to indicate the incidence of the particular combination of block and prolongation stammers found here. However, given that some adult stammerers do suffer from repetition, and that others may exhibit either block or prolongation alone, one may safely assume a figure considerably less than 1.0%. Further, when one considers that, among those sharing the block/prolongation combination, there will be variation in terms of their typical consonantal timings, then the degree and type of similarity established across the samples in this case can be seen as highly significant. Indeed, it was in view of this point of similarity, together with a further pathological tendency to misplace tonic syllables, a close match in pitch averages (103 Hz known sample; 104 Hz disputed sample) and other tight correspondences at both segmental and supra-segmental levels, that I was able to provide a firm opinion that the speech in the disputed sample was produced by the suspect.

Measurements of 'frequency structure'
The lung air upon which speech is produced does not only vibrate at the rate of vocal cord movement. There are vibrations at other, higher frequencies too, which are caused by the air 'rubbing' against the surfaces of the vocal organs and resonating in particular ways within the speech tract.

In the case of vowels these vibrations at higher frequencies are termed *formants*. Figures 3.6 and 3.7 show a spectrogram of two vowels /i:/ and /æ/.

The horizontal axis reflects time, and the vertical axis frequency. The calibrating lines represent frequency divisions of 1000 Hz (one kilohertz, or KHz). The dark bars are the formants. Thus, for example, we can see that for /i:/ the lowest formant (known as 'f1') is around 200 Hz and the next one (f2) is a little over 2 KHz. For /æ/ f1 is around 800 Hz and f2 occurs at about 1.5 KHz.

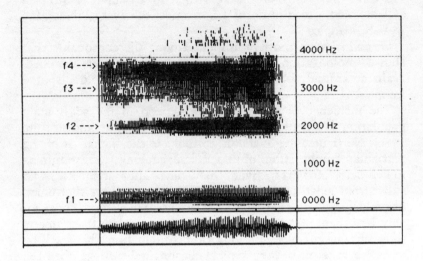

Figure 3.6 Spectrogram of /i:/ indicating formant positions

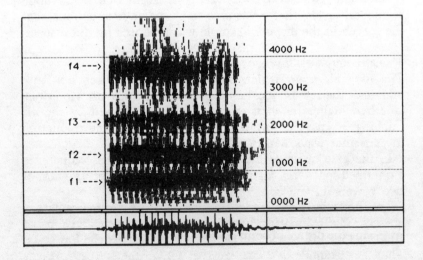

Figure 3.7 Spectrogram of /æ/ indicating formant positions

It is the occurrence of formants at different frequencies which is responsible for giving vowels their different qualities.

In the earlier North American tradition of forensic speaker identification (cf. Kersta, 1962), great stress was placed upon the comparison of spectrograms of the known and disputed samples. The concept behind this is that, just as spectrographic differences can be identified between the various vowel and consonant phonemes, so such differences will be apparent between different speakers' pronunciations of them. Early work in the USA held out great hopes for this use of spectrograms, and people, in my view, prematurely and often irresponsibly, began to talk about 'voice-printing', placing the work of the forensic phonetician on a par with that of the finger-print examiner. Subsequent research has shown this idea to be flawed.

In comparing speech samples, I do make use of spectrograms to examine formant configurations, and in some cases these can be of assistance in arriving at an opinion. Figures 3.8 and 3.9 represent two spectrograms of the suspect and a caller to the fire service in an arson case saying the words 'right-hand side'. In this case there was overwhelming evidence of other kinds that the suspect was, in fact, the caller, and one can observe close correspondences between the spectrograms.

Speakers' hesitation markers ('ums', 'ers') merit special attention when comparing samples. Although there is regionally and socially based variation in the realisation of the markers, there is also a very great deal of individual variation within geographical regions and social groups. Moreover, there is evidence that many individuals are highly consistent in their realisations (Künzel, 1987).

Realisations I have recorded as occurring within Received Pronunciation range from front, central and back monophthongs with varying degrees of openness (e.g. [e::], [ɛ::], [ə::], [a::]) to opening, closing and centring diphthongs (e.g. [əa̲], [ɛe], [aə]). All of these variants may or may not be completed with a bilabial nasal, e.g. [ə:m], [a:m].

Spectrography provides a convenient and accurate means of assessing the degree of comparability between hesitation markers from different speech samples. Figures 3.10 and 3.11 are of hesitation markers taken from the known and disputed speech samples in the same arson case as Figures 3.8 and 3.9. The similarity of formant configurations is once more readily apparent.

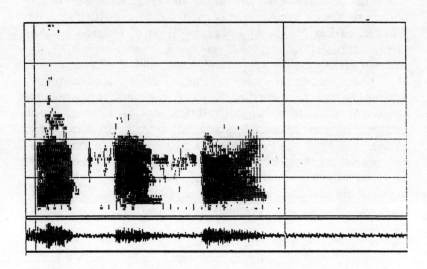

Figure 3.8 Spectrogram of words 'right-hand side' from criminal telephone call

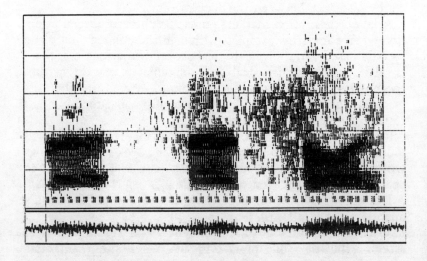

Figure 3.9 Spectrogram of words 'right-hand side' (expanded time base) spoken by suspect

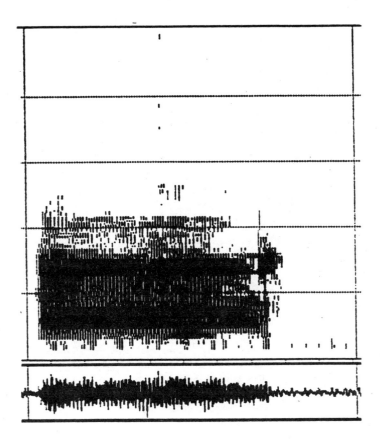

Figure 3.10 Spectrogram of hesitation marker from criminal
telephone call

Leaving aside the feature of hesitation markers, spectrography
cannot be regarded as a certain way of determining whether two
speech samples of speech are of a common source. Spectrograms
of the same word rendered by the same person can look very
different. Also, spectrograms of the same word spoken by
different people may look very similar. In a recent case of
murder, the killer made a telephone call to the ambulance
service reporting the injuries to his victim. The call was
recorded and transcribed. The suspect and six policemen of
similar age and social and regional background read aloud from
the transcripts and had their voices recorded. Spectrograms
revealed only very broad resemblances between the speech of

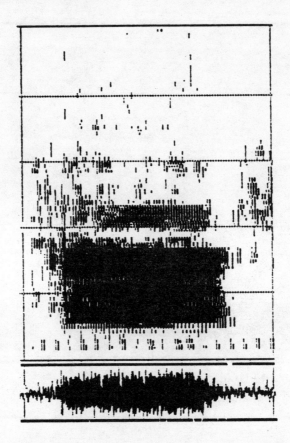

Figure 3.11 Spectrogram of hesitation marker used by suspect

the suspect and that of the caller. Those of samples taken from
two of the policemen, however, provided extremely tight
matches.

Undoubtedly, the examination of vowel formant configurations is a valuable tool in the overall battery available to the
forensic phonetician, and in certain cases it has provided very
important evidence (see Nolan, in press). However, this aspect
of spectrography must be used judiciously, in combination with
other acoustic and auditory methods. Further, as explained later
in this chapter, its use may be very dangerous outside the hands
of the skilled phonetician.

Voice quality
At the risk of oversimplifying, 'voice quality' is the term used to refer to the combination of resonances upon which the stream of speech is 'overlaid'. One might find two individuals who pronounced each of the vowel and consonant sounds in a very similar way, who had very closely matched pitch averages, pitch ranges and intonation patterns, but, who, nevertheless, sounded very different from one another. One speaker might be heard as having, say, a 'nasalised' voice and the other an 'adenoidal' voice; one voice could be heard as 'creaky', the other as 'breathy', and so on. These are just a few of the more accessible labels phoneticians have used to describe voice quality (Laver, 1980).

Voice quality is recognised as varying quite widely across individual speakers. Many variations are physiologically caused. They arise from differences in the size, shape and relative proportions of certain speech organs and the various 'resonating chambers' within the vocal tract. Most of the auditory impressions brought about by these differences are very difficult to quantify. And, in the majority of instances, spectrographic examinations of samples are not of great assistance to the forensic phonetician in this respect. The reason for this is that most of the significant information about voice quality is carried by the third and fourth formants, and in most cases at least one of the samples one is comparing has been recorded over a telephone line. Telephone lines are responsive to frequencies up to around 3-3.4 KHz, and in speech obtained over the telephone the higher formants are often missing, or, at best, poorly represented.

One aspect of voice quality which can be examined instrumentally, though not by spectrography, is that known as *laryngealisation*, or *glottal creak*. This is the 'gravelly' effect particularly associated with the voices of mature men when they are speaking in the lower part of their pitch range. It is produced by holding closed the glottis at one end, thus allowing vibration only at the other. In these circumstances the air escapes as a series of small 'pops', at a lower frequency than normal voice.

Research in which I am presently engaged is showing that speakers vary widely in terms of the point in their pitch range at which they 'descend' into glottal creak, and also in terms of the point at which they 'ascend' out of it into normal voice. Results to date also indicate that the transition points in and out of creak are relatively constant for individuals. It is anticipated that measures of creak transition will be added to the existing battery of tests available to the forensic phonetician.

The necessity for auditory phonetic analysis

So far in this chapter I have made a case for the use of instrumental analyses of speech samples, and have outlined some specific features of speech that can profitably be examined by instrumental means. It should be made clear that the instrumental tests set out here cannot provide a 'stand-alone' alternative to detailed auditory examinations of the types described in other chapters. The instrumental work is intended to complement the auditory examinations, not to replace them. Indeed, as I indicated above, without the support of detailed analyses undertaken by a properly trained and experienced auditory phonetician, the results of instrumental examinations can be dangerously misleading. This becomes apparent from a consideration of the following two cases.

The first is a case of arson. Shortly after the firing of a church in a West Lancashire town, a 999 call was received by the fire brigade reporting, among other things, that the caller could see 'a fire coming from the side of the church'. A lecturer in acoustics acted as an expert in speaker identification for the defence and made instrumental measurements of various aspects of this phrase as it appeared in a recording of the 999 call and in a controlled recording of the suspect reading aloud from a transcript of the call. Among other differences between the two samples he noted from an instrumental analysis that in respect of the construction 'fire coming', 'the caller's waveform has a decaying envelope [i.e. a feature indicating decreasing amplitude] for the /r/ whereas [the suspect's] does not'. Whilst some Lancashire accents do preserve /r/ in non-prevocalic environments, both samples in this case were entirely non-rhotic. There was no /r/ consonant at the end of the word 'fire'. The expert believed he was comparing /r/ consonants, but the segments in question were, in fact, the final schwa elements of the triphthong /aɪə/!

The second case is one of blackmail. A sound engineer claiming expertise in speaker identification undertook a comparison of speech samples and wrote a report for the defence. The expert failed quite systematically to identify instances of vowel reduction. Indeed, one suspects that he was wholly unaware of the relationships between vowel quality and syllable stress, even at the level of theory. The word 'problem', which occurred five times in the course of a criminal telephone call, was mistranscribed as containing the vowel phoneme /e/ rather than /ə/ in the unstressed syllable. The expert produced a series of very elegantly presented spectrograms in demonstration of his conclusion that the suspect 'could not possibly have made the telephone call'. The spectrographic comparisons were of the suspect's /e/ vowel taken from the words 'letter' and 'better' placed alongside the caller's rendering of 'the same vowel' taken from the second syllable of each of the five productions of the word 'problem'. They had, in the words of the expert, 'very different formant structures'.

The point arising from these examples is, I think, obvious: whilst auditory phonetic analysis alone may be limited in the respects that I have outlined, it is, nevertheless, the fundamental component, the absolute cornerstone of the forensic comparison. Without basic skills of auditory phonetic analysis, one may well be led into making instrumental comparisons of entirely non-comparable elements of speech across the known and disputed samples. The danger of forming a conclusion on the basis of such comparisons cannot be over-emphasised.

The most reliable opinions on speaker identity are in my view likely to be those founded upon both auditory and acoustic tests.

Determination of disputed utterances

As stated at the outset of this chapter, evidential tape recordings may also be challenged on the ground that words spoken have been wrongly heard and transcribed. There are two main factors which give rise to disputes over what was said.

The first is the poor quality recording. A good many of the recordings submitted as legal evidence are of poor sound quality. The problems encountered are very often caused by high levels of background sound, telephone line noise, static interference, and so on. The difficulties of interpreting speech overlaid with noise are in some cases made worse by weak recording signals.

A sizeable proportion of the work carried out in my own laboratory consists of attempting to 'enhance' the sound quality of recordings by suppressing unwanted noise, using various kinds of sound filter. The success of sound filtering techniques in this respect is entirely dependent upon the nature of the interfering noise. If the problem noise is a relatively discrete tone, high frequency 'hiss' or low frequency 'rumble', then sound filtering can often do a great deal to improve the intelligibility of the questioned words. If, however, the noise occupies a wide frequency band, and substantially overlaps with that responsible for carrying the speech signal, sound filtering techniques can make little improvement. Any attempt to suppress the unwanted noise suppresses the speech signal, too.

In these cases, I have developed an alternative method for clarifying what was said. This involves having available a better quality and more extensive sample of speech from the speaker in the disputed section of the evidential recording. An auditory study, involving narrow phonetic transcriptions and notes on such features as speech rhythms, patterns of elision and assimilation, is made of the speech in the reference sample. Equipped with knowledge of the speaker's phonology, the phonetician is then in a position of advantage when it comes to re-appraising the unclear words. In cases where I have applied this method, the court has been prepared to admit my interpretation of the disputed words as expert testimony.

The second type of case where the words spoken become subject to legal dispute involves speech patterns which are unfamiliar to the person responsible for making the court transcription. Here one might include pathological speech and various foreign and regional accents.

In cases of this kind in which I have acted, the quality of the recording has not been problematic, and here it has been possible to undertake acoustic as well as auditory phonetic examinations of the disputed and reference samples.

One such case involved a doctor of Greek extraction who spoke English with a strong Greek accent. He had been tape-recorded in his surgery providing controlled drugs in tablet form to a man posing as a drug addict. On handing the man the prescription, he was recorded saying 'you can/can't inject those things'. In a disciplinary tribunal the prosecution held that the ambiguous word was 'can' and that the doctor was acting irresponsibly in recommending that his patient grind up tablets for injection. The defence argued that the word was 'can't', and that the doctor was, in fact, acting responsibly in warning the patient against a dangerous practice.

At the request of the defence I examined the disputed utterance, and also a sample of conversation involving the doctor where he used the words 'can' and 'can't' several times. Initial auditory examinations of the reference sample revealed that the doctor typically elided the final /t/ of 'can't', thus leaving 'can' and 'can't' with the same consonant-vowel-consonant structure. They also indicated that the doctor used a front vowel in both 'can' and 'can't', and that his vowel in 'can' was pronounced with a tongue position only slightly higher than that he used in 'can't'.

Spectrographic examinations of the reference samples showed the first formant of his 'can' vowel to be lower and the second formant higher than those of his 'can't' vowel. The formant values of the vowel in the disputed word fell clearly within the range associated with his 'can't' vowel and outside those associated with his 'can'. On the basis of these findings, I was able to provide an opinion to the tribunal in support of the defence case.

There have been several cases of this kind where instrumental examinations have been of great assistance in the formation of an opinion. As with cases of speaker identification, my own view is that a combination of instrumental and auditory methods is likely to provide the best way forward.

Authentication of recordings

The third type of dispute which may arise with regard to evidential recordings involves the claim that the recording represents an edited version of what was said, certain words and utterances having been deleted, inserted out of context or otherwise re-arranged, in order, for example, to discredit a defendant or witness.

The most significant developments in methods for detecting evidence of editing on audio recordings have been made by sound engineers, rather than phoneticians, and my own forensic casework in tape authentication now includes these techniques.

However, in authenticating a tape recording of conversation the first examinations I normally carry out are auditory phonetic ones. That is not to say that the entire conversation is transcribed phonetically, but that it is examined in short sections. Each section is subjected to detailed analytic listening whilst being repeated many times on a tape machine with a loopback facility. The listening is informed by research knowledge of the phonology of natural conversation. The set of features one is listening for includes unexpected or unexplained shifts in the pitch of speakers' voices and foreshortening of vowel or consonant sounds, as may occur when sections of speech have been deleted from or inserted into an edited recording.

If 'unnatural' patterns are detected, the relevant section of the recording is subjected to acoustic tests, in order to provide instrumental corroboration of the auditory judgments.

The authentication techniques deriving from sound engineering currently in use include acoustic and micrographic examination of switching transients and of the recording more generally. However, many of these tests are applied only in the event of the basic phonetic examinations having revealed suspicious features. In this sense, then, the phonetic examinations - auditory and instrumental - are fundamental to work in this area.

Conclusion

In this chapter I have attempted to provide an introduction to a wider range of forensic applications of phonetics. Throughout, I have stressed the role of acoustic as well as auditory phonetic analysis in the various fields of forensic phonetic investigation. The description of the methods used has, by necessity, been less than complete, a full understanding of what is involved being dependent upon prior detailed knowledge of phonetics - something which is not assumed in the reader.

It is certain that in ten years from now the range of methods included in a chapter of this sort would be more extensive than that set out here. As a subject discipline, phonetics is a comparative newcomer to forensic enquiry, and techniques are developing rapidly, on the basis of ongoing research. For various theoretical reasons, I cannot foresee a day when phoneticians will be able to identify a speaker with the degree of certainty associated with the matching of finger-prints or DNA profiles. However, it is equally certain that the degree of reliability one may attach to the opinions of the forensic phonetician will be increased in respect of each of the areas discussed here, and that many of the improvements will arise from acoustically-based research studies.

Chapter 4

Aspects of Forensic Phonetics

There are many ways in which phonetics can be of use in the forensic context, and I think phoneticians would be in general agreement if I said that those ways fall into two broad categories, with a number of sub-categories. I would like to make it clear at this point that I am not, in suggesting these divisions of the field, attempting to set up hermetic boundaries, but simply breaking up what is in fact a very complex field for the sake of ease of access and discussion.

The first of the two broad categories includes those situations in which the police, for example, are carrying out their preliminary investigations with, probably, no particular suspects in mind. They will typically be in possession of a speech sample of some kind, such as a copy of a telephone call involving an unknown speaker, or a cassette recorded by an unknown person. Here the investigators will obviously be helped by any information the phonetician can give them with respect to the unknown speaker's background. Such cases constitute the 'investigative' or 'intelligence' category, and can be listed under four headings. We will return to these headings in more detail in a moment.

The second category in which phonetics can be of use involves those cases where the investigators have advanced matters to a more specific target, usually in the form of specific suspects, although other targets are possible, as I shall explain in due course. In my experience this category, which we might call the 'evidential', accounts for the vast majority of cases, and we will, in consequence, devote most time to a consideration of its many aspects, and in some detail. Before embarking on that topic, though, let us return briefly to the investigative category, and a consideration of the kinds of situation in which phonetics has been of assistance in building up a picture of an unknown person on the basis of his speech.

Probably the first and most obvious thing investigators might want to know about an unknown speaker is: 'Where does he come from?' George Bernard Shaw took considerable literary licence in portraying the abilities of Professor Higgins in *Pygmalion* as, really, superhuman in the matter of *accent location*, and his is the responsibility for the vastly inflated expectations investigators sometimes have of ordinary, human phoneticians in this direction. Courts, too, are not exempt from such misapprehensions, and both there and in the media the phonetician can occasionally find himself, to his embarrassment, credited with phonetic capacities he simply does not possess. Though considerably more modest in their claims than Shaw's fictional character, phoneticians with the appropriate experience and expertise can achieve some very impressive results; Stanley Ellis and Jack Windsor-Lewis of Leeds University, as well as Peter French for example, have carried out accent location exercises which have proved invaluable to the progress of the cases they were consulted on.

Any phonetician involved in accent location will gladly acknowledge the importance of the intuitive 'feel' for a local as opposed to a non-local accent which an accent-conscious layman may have. It is certainly true that human beings vary considerably in their auditory attention and memory, so that a speech event, for example, which would pass one person by, leaving no trace in his auditory memory and exciting no reaction, would strike another as noteworthy in some way, perhaps in the matter of accent, and he would retain an accurate auditory impression of that speech event. The world abounds with natural phoneticians, but it might lead to serious difficulties if courts were to accept any given layman's assurance that he was one of them. The opinion of a trained phonetician would be indispensable in any reliable assessment of natural phoneticians. I think it would probably be true to say that, of all the phonetician's skills, accent location remains the one of greatest interest and perhaps even slightly romantic attraction to the layman, and this is only partly attributable to G.B. Shaw's hyperbole.

In cases of accent location the unknown speech sample is assumed to be genuine, and the phonetician's task is to identify the regional origin of the speaker. The layman often refers to the speaker's birthplace, as if that in itself were of some significance in determining the speaker's accent. If we were born speaking this might be so, but since we are not, it is clearly the speaker's upbringing and subsequent associations which are of relevance; I do not believe that any modern academic would seriously want to propose a theory of genetically-determined regional accent.

In cases falling under the heading of *counterfeit accent* there is some reason to suspect that the speaker's accent as heard in the recording might not be their usual one. There are many reasons why a speaker might want to conceal his/her identity by adopting an accent which is not their own: people making telephone calls for the purposes of extorting money, kidnappers, terrorists, obscene callers speaking to someone who would probably recognise their undisguised speech, etc., etc.

One case which I dealt with in this category related to a cassette-tape sent to a police force which had just arrested two suspects on strong evidence of their having caused explosions. The caller gave what purported to be a 'confession' of his involvement in an aspect of the crime attributed to the arrested men, assuring the police that these young men could not, therefore, have been involved. The sample extended to several pages of transcript, since the level of detailed information required lengthy exposition if it was to be convincing. The accent, on first hearing, seemed to be a mixture of some kind of Scottish with a general north-east English type. Closer attention, however, revealed the presence of two very indicative things; firstly there were occasional traces of a third accent, and secondly there was very considerable, one might even say wild variation in the pronunciation of the same phoneme, even in the same word, and this sometimes in the same sentence. For example, the speaker produced the word: 'car' three times in the same sentence, the first time with a vowel quality close to that of Cardinal Vowel 5, i.e. open and back, the second time with a quality between CV4 and CV5, i.e. open and central, and the third time with a quality very close to that of CV4, but raised above open. It became clear to me that such extreme variation would be highly unlikely in any sort of natural accent - certainly it was well outside my experience in that direction. It seemed much more likely that the speaker was putting on these features in order to conceal his real accent. And I felt the most likely candidate for the role of his real accent was the one which showed only rare traces, being usually obscured by the intentionally distracting character of his assumed accent. There were three particular features of the obscured accent that I noticed: a tense, close, spread vowel in word-final position, e.g. 'only'; a level diphthong (i.e. with both elements of equal prominence) with a close, back, rounded final quality, as in '*due*' and lengthening of intervocalic consonants, as in '*office*'. Although these features did not occur on every theoretically possible occasion, they did, when taken together with a number of other, principally vowel features, present a reasonable picture of a particular accent-type. Whilst my conclusions here were far from being in the 'Professor Higgins' league, I was able to state within a fairly broad approximation where I thought the speaker to have come from, i.e. South Wales. Within the context of that particular case, that intelligence was very helpful. I subsequently learnt that my input to the case had made it possible for the police to pursue their enquiries in the right direction, and that a conviction had eventually been secured.

Obviously my job here was made a lot easier by the very long sample – if the speaker had been able to get his message across in only a few words he might have succeeded in deceiving the listener. However, in the very nature of things such messages usually do require considerable elaboration, with its inevitable concomittant danger, from the would-be deceiver's point of view, of making a mistake. The phonetician, of course, has no remedy against the perfect accent-imitator, in the same way as any perfect counterfeit will elude detection, but perfection in the phonetics area seems, fortunately, to be very rare. Even professional imitators have been known to make mistakes in extended samples, whilst the amateur, I think, usually does let his accent slip.

Hybrid accent. Here again the accent appears to be genuine, but contains features which are rare within the speech of one person. One case I dealt with in this category involved a telephone call to a government office of a Mediterranean country threatening to release a highly toxic substance in that country during the tourist season unless a considerable ransom were paid. The caller was a youngish male with what was almost totally a London accent. Two characteristics were decidedly not of a London type though; one was a particularly close front vowel at the ends of words like 'only', which would normally be found in relatively few accents, such as Liverpool, South Wales and Newcastle-on-Tyne; the other was a modification of certain consonant sounds at the ends of words/syllables when followed immediately by certain other consonants. This feature is usually described as: anticipatory assimilation of voice, and involves the changing of voiceless sounds such as /p/, /t/ and /k/ to their voiced equivalents: /b/, /d/ and /g/ when they occur at the end of a word/syllable, and are followed without a pause by a voiced consonant such as: /b/, /d/, /g/. A shibboleth for this kind of process is the word 'football', which is pronounced by very many people in or from the North East of England as 'foodball' (without, of course, affecting the vowel qualities). This kind of assimilation is otherwise very rare amongst native speakers of English. It is not recorded either on Merseyside or in South Wales. Certain people irrespective of region might also be heard to do it when drunk, but that would be for entirely different reasons, of course!

It is, as it happens, very common in the English of speakers whose native language is one of the very many in which it occurs. This would include any from the Romance group, such as French and Romanian, or the Slavonic group, such as Polish and Russian, as well as a considerable list in which both Hungarian and Greek are to be found. The finer details of the caller's speech were of such a character that he must have been brought up in London – it is, quite simply, impossible for a foreign speaker without this kind of upbringing to acquire these features to that degree of perfection. I was, then, left with only two possibilities: one, that the speaker was a Londoner with two features from a regional English accent very distant in origin from London, or, much more likely in any case, but even more so given the present population make-up of London, that the caller was indeed a native London speaker (bearing in mind the meaning of 'native' in the context of accents discussed above), but with a family background in one of the non-English speech communities. Unfortunately, the accent features did not permit me to specify which of the foreign communities the investigators should look in, but when I reported my findings to the Anti-Terrorist Branch of New Scotland Yard, I was told that they had other reasons for thinking that the man might know Greek very well. In due course I learnt that a man of Greek Cypriot family background, but brought up in London, had been charged with the offence. I read subsequently that he had been brought to trial and found guilty.

The final heading in the investigative category of forensic phonetics is that of *special features*. This is a rather amorphous set of features which do not really find a home in any of the categories yet established. One of the most obvious speech characteristics to be included here is that of 'speech defect'. This term is usually self-explanatory, and misunderstandings by the layman are rare. Phoneticians will all have their own favourite examples of cases where such misunderstandings have occurred; I will content myself with mentioning the case of the middle-class mother with social aspirations for herself and her children who took her elder son, who had recently entered a state primary school in London to a speech therapist to have his newly-acquired 'speech defect' treated. Having listened for some minutes, in growing bafflement, to the child's speech, the therapist finally confessed to the mother that he had not been able to discern any evidence of a speech defect. The mother looked scornfully at him and exclaimed: 'But you must have noticed his ghastly Cockney accent!'

Genuine speech defects, of course, have an anatomical or a psychological explanation, often both. There are many sources of information on such defects, and since they are not part of the main area of this book I shall say no more on them, beyond observing that one would suppose, according to a superficial logic at least, that anyone with a speech defect would not get involved in any aspect of crime where their speech is likely to be recorded, such as making hoax telephone calls to the emergency services, and so on. On the contrary though, and very sadly, a disproportionately large number of such speakers do seem to get mixed up in that sort of thing, certainly on the basis of my experience. Clearly the speech defects of such people form only one aspect of more general personality problems, problems which the present serious and ongoing shortage of speech therapists in Britain is certainly not helping to alleviate.

Other features which might be added here include phonetic indices of the speaker's age and social background. Again, a good many things might be quoted here, but I shall limit myself to one of Peter French's examples. There is, it seems, an age split in popular Bristol speech, in that the youngest generation of speakers have adopted a characteristic of popular London speech – a prestige accent to them in a way that it was not to older generations in Bristol. The youngest generation, therefore, pronounces 'th' sounds in the London manner 'dis fing', whereas older generations of Bristolians produce and produced 'th' sounds as in RP, i.e. with dental fricatives. It is not, of course, the case that young Bristolians have suddenly lost the ability to produce the sounds, but rather that they are identifying with a different target, which is for them achieved by pronouncing differently words in which 'th' sounds occur.

In many of the cases I have described above, it is obvious that any success the phonetician might have had in contributing to the investigative process must have depended on a very detailed knowledge of a particular accent, or indeed of more than one accent. It would probably be no exaggeration to say that such detailed information is simply not available for many areas and communities in Britain, and that phoneticians' ability to help in any given case is, therefore, subject to the luck of the draw.

It is now appropriate to turn again to the evidential category of forensic phonetics, and here too to sub-divide the area. I would like to suggest the following headings:

- disputed utterances
- editing
- speaker-identification.

Under the first heading one typically finds a disagreement over the wording of a transcript - i.e. the details of what someone has said, or is alleged to have said in a given conversation. It is quite common, in cases involving tape-recorded conversations for example, to find the 'speaker-attribution' of the transcripts queried. The phonetician's task here is to compare in detail the disputed utterance with the attested utterances of each participant in the conversation, and to offer an opinion as to which, if any, was likely to have made that utterance. A typical case would be where the prosecution wishes to attribute a particular, incriminating utterance to a defendant, whilst the defence, for obvious reasons, wishes to attribute it either to some other, specific person, or to anybody in general, so long as it is not their client. I was present in court on one such occasion, where defence contended that a particular utterance had not been made by their client, but by some other person. Their difficulty in convincing the jury of the possibility of this lay in the fact that the conversation in question had been recorded during a car journey; three other men were present in the car, and the utterance did not sound remotely like any of them; furthermore, defence were unable to suggest how a fifth man had contrived firstly to join the car during its uninterrupted passage, secondly, to contribute to the conversation without having attracted the attention of the four men already there, and thirdly, to leave the car again before the end of the journey! The jury brought in a verdict of guilty, and were, therefore, clearly unimpressed with counsel's arguments on behalf of his client.

On some occasions the disputed material amounts to only one word or one syllable – usually something like: 'a statement' versus 'the statement' versus 'your statement'. Here the phonetician's experience in listening to speech events of very short duration is of great value, together with his background knowledge of the kind of phonetic effects the juxtaposition of different speech sounds is likely to produce. When speech sounds are placed together in speech, whether in isolated words or in connected utterances, one sound inevitably affects those next to or near it, something that the non-phonetician generally neither knows nor suspects.

The second heading is that of editing; this in its turn can be sub-divided into more precise groups, but they all have in common the factor that artificial changes are alleged to have been made in tape-recorded samples. Where digital recording techniques have been used, any editing can be done in such a way as to render it impossible to detect; most people who might want to edit tapes for the purposes of deception, however, do not command the financial and technical resources required for this kind of operation, and they are therefore limited to the relatively primitive techniques of the pre-computer age. Most people have read something about, but few seem really to have grasped the significance of, the vast expenditure of time, expertise and money which made the 'Watergate' tape-editing possible, and to allege, as is often done by defendants, that the police in their local station have carried out such operations is to push wishful thinking beyond any reasonable limit!

In principle one can have editing in, editing out and order-changing of sections of the tape. I have often been consulted on this particular subject, but so far I have never actually come across cases where any such editing has taken place – it does in fact seem to be something imported either from the world of high-level skulduggery, such as the Watergate affair, or from the realms of fiction. If the latter, we can hardly blame Shaw again. Other kinds of editing have produced results, i.e. false conversations, which I have encountered in actual cases. The theoretical possibilities here are: a conversation could be concocted by taking recorded natural utterances from, say, two people and joining those utterances into a new, spurious conversation; the utterances of both parties to the conversation could be read from prepared scripts and presented as natural conversation for the purposes of deception, or a combination of both methods could be used, in which one party's utterances derive from actual speech and the other's from a reading from a prepared script. I have been for some time involved in a case where, basically, the latter methods have been used, I believe, to produce a false conversation.

The alleged conversation involves two men speaking on a financial topic. They appear, superficially, to be relaxed, simply chatting at what sounds like a cocktail party. The conversation appears to resolve certain matters to the advantage of speaker A, let us call him, and speaker B is not now in a position to refute the claims of A. Towards the end of the conversation recording a third person, apparently somebody at the party, approaches the men and addresses a remark to them, which, of course, greatly enhances the impression of genuineness of the conversation as a whole.

I carried out an analysis of the intonation features of the speech of A and B as heard in the conversation. A number of interesting things emerged. First, the intonation patterns of A seemed very exaggerated, both in the matter of their overall pitch range and in the number of words in any given sentence which he selected for special emphasis, i.e. focus. Such over-emphasis is typical of the way in which some adults speak to children, foreigners or others they consider their intellectual inferiors. It is also heard from actors who are not very good and are trying too hard to sound 'real'.

Second, although the speech of B proved to be of an entirely natural character, when his responses were matched in their intonation to the leading questions of A, they were found to be incongruous – they did not hold up as natural answers to the questions they were purported to respond to. It seemed clear to me that the conversation was false, and that it had never taken place as a single event. Speaker A was clearly reading his part of the conversation sentence by sentence, with the later editing in of the utterances of B, which themselves had been edited out of at least one genuine conversation in which B had been involved. The crowning *tour de force* in this highly ingenious multi-recording operation was the superimposition of the conversation of A and B on to the background recording of the cocktail party in such a way as to synchronise the speech of the third person with the end of the A/B conversation.

From what I have already said concerning the cost of editing operations, it will be obvious that A, as the instigator of this attempted deception, must have commanded enormous resources, both of money and technical know-how. One of the main reasons for its failure was something quite simple, which no amount of financial outlay could have bought him however: elementary skill as an actor.

Let us now turn to the principal way in which phoneticians function in the forensic area - speaker-identification - and examine this complex topic in some detail.

Speaker-identification involves the comparison of samples of speech, and these are almost always tape-recorded. I have carried out comparisons in which one sample was live, whilst the other was recorded, usually surreptitiously, but these have always been in exceptional circumstances, where no other course of action was possible because of a policy of non-cooperation operated by the suspect. Live comparisons are, obviously, not very desirable because they eliminate some of the phonetician's principal aids - the facility to repeat a given passage, or to pause at a particular point in order to let one's short-term memory process the last phonetic event, and so on. These not particularly sophisticated facilities provided by the tape-recorder have, in fact, given the whole field of forensic phonetics its start; it can hardly have come into being without them.

I mentioned above the matter of tape-recorded speech samples being acquired surreptitiously, and perhaps a few words on that topic might be appropriate. In my experience it always has been, and apparently still is entirely unpredictable whether a given police force will make such recordings of suspects or not. It is a moral issue, one involving basic human rights, and many deputy chief constables take the view that to make such recordings would constitute an unacceptable infringement of those rights. They clearly feel that the right to privacy is fundamental, and one not lightly to be interfered with. Whilst agreeing that they are basically right, and that their moral stance is highly commendable, I must admit that my priorities are rather different. I believe there are many situations in which the making of covert recordings is vital to the investigative process, but the decision to carry it out must be shown to be justified by the investigators' assessment of the seriousness of the offence on any particular occasion. Obviously, discretion, goodwill and common-sense should play an active role when any such decisions are being made, and I would certainly not be happy to see an unchecked proliferation of the use of such techniques.

The following case is, I think, one which illustrates the valid use of concealed tape-recorders. I was recently consulted as phonetics expert by Her Majesty's Customs and Excise in a major VAT fraud investigation. Here most of the evidence took the form of such surreptitious recordings, both as to the participants in the fraud and their methods. Whilst the subsequent interviews of the suspects were recorded with their knowledge, they could not, obviously, have been informed about the recording of their conspiratorial meeting.

Many suspects give their consent to the now usual practice of interview-recording, whereby a double recording is made, and the suspect has access to one of the resulting cassettes. In this situation many suspects simply answer 'No comment' to any question put to them by the interviewers; I have even heard this answer given to formal questions relating to such already-established facts as their names, date of birth, address, etc., which must sorely tax the patience of the interviewers! In my experience they usually handle such complications with exemplary forbearance.

I have known quite a few instances where an extra, unofficial recording has been made of pre- and/or post-interview conversation with the suspect when they are expected to behave in an obstructive manner in the interview proper, for example, by refusing to talk at all, or by repeating 'No comment'. Clearly, any number of repetitions of this phrase cannot constitute a speech sample which would be of any use in a speaker-identification exercise, whereas the surreptitious recording has often yielded useful material. Once again, I take the purely practical view that such a sample is better than none at all.

When one is speaking of civil rights, one must also take into account the right of members of the public not to be robbed, defrauded, or otherwise offended against by people whose only understanding of 'civil rights' is the right to get away with as much as they can, and to use any defence they can devise in the event of their being caught, including claims of 'foul play' by the forces of the law. Their sudden conversion to belief in legality and equity would be moving if it were genuine, and not merely a subterfuge. There are constraints on the making of covert recordings, and if there were any irregularity in the ways in which they had been obtained, it would certainly be possible for counsel to argue that they should be ruled inadmissible. I have never actually been involved in a case in which a speech-sample was rejected by a judge because it had been obtained secretly, although this remains an ever-present possibility. It should be remembered, too, as my own experience has shown on dozens of occasions, that suspects can be eliminated from enquiries on the basis of such recordings; one must consider the very real right of a person to be removed from suspicion at the earliest possible stage of an enquiry. If they are not thus removed, they are very likely to suffer unnecessary and prolonged distress.

Let us proceed on the assumption that the phonetician has been supplied with a number of tape-recorded speech samples, and that he will not be exercised as to how those samples were obtained. His first job is to play through all the samples in order to assess their acceptability as such. It is, for example, by no means unknown for one or some of the samples to be quite unsuitable for analysis because their quality is so poor that not enough of the speech material can be heard in order to build up a viable sample for comparison purposes. When this occurs it is sometimes possible electronically to enhance the quality of the recording. (More has been said on this in Chapter 3.) In the past, judges were very often unhappy about this operation, because it was argued that the process changed the character of an item of evidence. They often, therefore, did not permit such processed recordings to be presented as evidence in court. I think it is the case now that judges, along with the rest of us, have developed greater familiarity with electronic technology, and accept that an enhanced recording is certainly not altered evidence. The phonetician giving evidence on the basis of such enhanced recordings would, however, always be well-advised to listen to and be prepared to present in court the non-enhanced copies, just to be on the safe side.

Where the matter of clarity is involved, it is worth remembering that this is not an absolute, but a subjective continuum, depending on, amongst other things, the listener's experience in dealing with tape-recorded samples. Many phoneticians, for example, do not work with any degree of regularity with recorded samples of natural speech, with all the problems that that entails, but rather with samples recorded under ideal circumstances in the studio. Such of my colleagues who do work in this way, and it is, of course, perfectly proper from an academic point of view that they should, find the average forensic recording rather daunting, in that they have difficulty in actually hearing what is going on in terms of the speech signal. Familiarity with forensic samples can be a considerable advantage in this matter, but it is not the deciding factor in determining whether a given listener, even a phonetician, will be able to extract the message from such recordings.

Another, but related factor which affects the subjective impression of clarity is that of auditory focus. This psychologically mysterious process enables the listener to focus his attention on, for example, a particular speaker, and to marginalise the distractions of other speakers and/or background noise in the context of a crowded and noisy party. We can all do this to a greater or lesser extent, and I am sure we can all think of situations in which we have not managed to do so, and not exclusively in the context of conversation, although this would constitute the major category of such occurrences. In the conversational situation I have usually failed to extract any message at all from the average airline pilot's intercom, whilst in the realm of musical performance for example, it seems to be quite common for a certain type of listener to be unable to marginalise the mechanical noise of the harpsichord, and consequently to hear only that noise and not the music! And I know the same to be true of other musical instruments in the playing of which there is an element of noise.

The term 'transcript' is used in the forensic context to refer to the orthographic version of a recorded speech sample, and this is, of course, quite different from a 'transcription' of that sample, which would be carried out using the symbols of the IPA. A trained phonetician would be responsible for the latter, and would not normally make a transcript of the sample if his only interest in it lay in some phonetic aspect, such as accent-location, and the supplier of the sample had made, or caused to be made, a transcript which the phonetician found adequate. When good transcripts are supplied, the phonetician can get on with the real substance of his work, and does not have to spend time on an unnecessary operation. Not all transcripts are adequate, though, a topic to which I shall return in a moment.

There are other occasions also when an employer feels happier with a transcript made by someone accustomed to listening to and deciphering recordings of unscripted speech. I have worked on many cases where the only requirement was for me to produce a better transcript than the one initially available; these have usually been for the defence. Naturally, on such occasions the hope is that I would produce a version of a less-incriminating character for their client. As it happens, I have never actually done so, but the possibility remains that on some future occasion I could, and this is a very real possibility if one takes into account the pretty abysmal quality of some transcripts.

Over the years I have received a very large number of transcripts which were decidedly inadequate, and this in a variety of ways. One oddity which has become less common, although still occurs from time to time, is the transcript from which all obscenities have been removed. In what I would assume to be the reader's own normal conversation that omission would probably not amount to very much, if, indeed, anything, but in the conversation of a certain type of criminal the omitted material could represent a substantial proportion of all the words spoken. It often happens that vital phonetic comparisons are made, and have to be made because there is no other usable sample, on the basis of obscene words.

The progressive diminution of such transcripts is, probably, due to a number of causes. For example, when such work was first carried out in police forces, it seemed to be the practice to hand the job over to a civilian typist, who, as often as not, was a young girl for whom the typing of obscenities would have caused acute embarrassment. The making of a good transcript, especially when the recordings are relatively noisy, and possibly more than one person is speaking, requires a high degree of skill, a particular aptitude which varies from person to person, and which is not related in any simple way to their experience in listening to difficult samples. It follows, then, that the job of making transcripts should be delegated to anyone who is good at it, irrespective of their status, and that it cannot simply be entrusted to the most junior member of the office. It seems that this principle is being acted upon in more and more cases.

Another reason for the change, it seems to me, could be that public attitudes to obscenities have changed drastically over the period of time that I have been involved in reading transcripts. With the status of such expressions on the radio, on television and in the theatre, as well as in pop music, having changed from impermissible to obligatory, it becomes more and more unlikely that anyone can be found who is actually embarrassed by them.

Some transcripts give the appearance of neatness and accuracy when one first reads them, in that all the sentences end properly, and all the utterances make sense. When one relates them, or rather, attempts to relate them to the recorded sample, however, there is little relationship between them – the transcript-writer has edited the conversation. To make everything tidy he had omitted anything which he did not understand, and has often joined the beginning of an uncompleted sentence to the end of a totally different sentence, the beginning of which he could not hear clearly enough. By this editing process the writer has, often enough, produced 'sentences' which mean the complete opposite of what was actually said. Under these circumstances the phonetician must make a new, corrected transcript, and this will be anything up to five times longer than the original transcript. If such an editing operation were carried out to the effect that the writer's own 'side' appeared to gain in the sense of incriminating evidence, one would be quite justified in concluding that, consciously or otherwise, the editing was done to that purpose. The fact of the matter is, though, that it seems to be entirely random as to whether the writer's side will gain or not, since such edited transcripts often appear to favour the opposing side, whereas the corrected version usually does not. It would be possible, I suppose, to suggest that the writer, if an employee of the police, Customs, etc., has the subconscious wish to undermine their case, with the further implication that his deeper motivations need to be explored by those qualified to do so. If one subscribes to the belief that there is no such thing as a superficial action, and that all apparently simple actions have underlying hidden and unwelcome explanations, then one must, indeed, carry out such an examination.

On a less sinister level, perhaps it is the case that the writer who unconsciously edits is simply the victim of his own inadequate auditory focus: he perceives such speech samples in an entirely superficial way, and does the best with what he can perceive. Writers who have this kind of problem with recorded material do not seem to have any difficulties in handling ordinary conversation, which serves to emphasise the special status of tape-recorded material for certain individuals. Needless to say, when someone has been discovered to have made such an edited transcript, they should not be entrusted with that task on any future occasion, no matter what the pressure may be on manpower resources. In the long run there will be an economy of time and money, because the phonetician will not have to re-write the transcript.

Fortunately, transcripts do have their funnier side. A transcript made of the speech of one of his friends in connection with the conspiracy case against a leading Liberal politician included the frequent occurrence of the word 'air', as in 'We must get together about this air', and so on. When I looked at the transcript I was baffled by this, because it did not appear to bear any kind of relationship to the subject-matter of the conversations in which it occurred. However, upon hearing the speaker on the tape, all became clear to me. The subject was a speaker of that socially-restricted sub-accent of RP which is customarily described as 'advanced' in the world of phonetics, i.e. a descriptive term. In the non-RP speaking layman's value judgment terminology, though, it would probably be identified as 'affected' or 'posh'. The speaker was, in fact, saying his equivalent of the hesitation noise, which, for most of us, would be represented orthographically with reasonable accuracy as 'er'. The above utterance was, in fact, his equivalent of the sentence: 'We must get together about this, er . . . '. Since this kind of pronunciation must have sounded quite exotic to the transcript writer, he interpreted what the speaker intended merely as a noise signalling: 'I am hesitating', as a lexical item, even though he could have made no more sense of the transcript when it was included in it than I could. In fact, in listening to some thousands of speech samples in the forensic context, I have only very occasionally come across this kind of hesitation noise. When it is used by a speaker, he is signalling not only that he is hesitating, but that he also belongs, or wishes the listener to assume that he belongs to a particularly elevated social stratum. The rarity of it in the forensic context is, conceivably, an indicator that people on that particular level of society do not get themselves recorded on tape in criminal investigations, either because they do not engage in criminal activities, or because they are worldly-wise enough to know how to avoid being recorded if they do.

Having followed up some of the implications of the question of clarity of samples, it is now appropriate for us to return to the second aspect of the adequacy of speech samples for forensic purposes: the actual speech content, i.e. how many words are there in the sample? This, too, is not an absolute, but is relative to the nature of the speaker's pronunciation and voice quality. If there are unusual features in either or both of these, such as a regularly mispronounced word or a speech defect, etc., the number of words that the phonetician would regard as adequate for his purposes would obviously be considerably reduced. On a number of occasions I have felt able to arrive at a very high level of positive identification on the basis of an X sample of only a few dozen words, where such idiosyncratic features were present. The absence of any such idiosyncracies would necessitate a larger body of words, and in such cases I would usually hope for something in the region of a hundred words as a sample permitting, potentially, the highest level of identification. Samples which are both short and lacking idiosyncracies would, obviously, produce at most some lower level of identification. Of course, there is no such thing as a sample which is too extensive – one would in principle always hope for the largest sample possible.

This latter point is of considerable importance to anyone finding themselves in a situation where they are, let us say, trying to get a sample from an unknown caller on the telephone, or from a suspect in an interview room, and so on. It has been my experience on more than one occasion that the person controlling the conversation has actually interrupted a speaker whose sample they knew was going to be required for comparison purposes, when that speaker had clearly embarked on a topic they felt they wanted to talk on at some length. The resulting samples have quite often not been adequate for comparison purposes because the subject has reacted by henceforth refusing to open up and speak in anything more than mumbled monosyllables; in such cases I have had to return tapes to the investigators with a note saying the samples were not adequate. The reason why such counter-productive situations arise is not difficult to work out. For the inexperienced interviewer, 'control' of a conversation is exerted in a relatively heavy manner, with what can superficially be mistaken for effective management of turn-taking, topic selection and so on. In other words, the controller does not allow the controlled to take the initiative in the conversation, and every time it looks as if he might be going to do so, he is brought up short by some appropriate technique applied by the controller. It should, I think, be remembered that control of a conversation cannot be treated as if it were an absolute, but must be related to the ultimate goal of the conversation. If that goal is to get the speaker to provide the longest sample of his speech that he can be prevailed upon to give, then that must take precedence over other, perhaps under different circumstances quite proper considerations, such as keeping the speaker to the point, not allowing him to waste time, etc., etc. From the phonetician's point of view, no utterance in a potential forensic sample is irrelevant, and no sample is too long. By appearing to give the subject his head, by seeming to lose control of the conversation in conventional terms at least, the controller is actually still in control, but on a subtler and, probably, ultimately more productive level.

Apart from members of the police, few people have occasion to put this kind of ability to the test, and even police officers do not necessarily get much practice at it. When such skills are needed there seems to be considerable variation in natural aptitude. I was consulted by a police force in the west of England on a very distressing series of anonymous obscene telephone calls. After a considerable number of these calls had been made, and a number of them recorded, a suspect was eventually suggested. It was necessary to obtain a sample of that suspect's speech, and because, in the judgment of the local police, he would not be likely to co-operate in giving one voluntarily, it was decided that an officer should telephone him on some fictitious but feasible topic, and that that call should be recorded. One officer tried, but with very little to show by way of usable sample. He clearly found it extremely difficult to lead the suspect into expressing himself fluently. Another officer tried, in a much more personal manner, and established good contact with the suspect, who then chatted for some time, and in a totally relaxed manner. The resulting sample was sent to me for comparison with the obscene calls, and I found considerable similarity between the samples. I duly reported this opinion to the police force, and the suspect was confronted with it. He admitted having made the obscene calls in question, and also confessed to having made some dozens of similar calls, many of which had not been reported.

Clearly some people are more skilful at this kind of acting, deception, call it what you will, than others. The first case I was involved in in which this was a major issue was in the south of England. A burglar had broken into the house of an elderly lady and stolen a valuable oil painting. Apparently not having an illicit buyer for the painting, and presumably finding it not to his personal taste and therefore not worth keeping for himself, the burglar telephoned the old lady and told her she would never see her painting again unless she were prepared to pay him a substantial sum of money to return it. He also told her that if she contacted the police he would automatically destroy the painting. Although naturally very distressed at this, coming as it did on top of the distress she already felt as a result of having her house burgled, she very wisely ignored his threats and made contact with her local police. They asked my advice as to how she should set about dealing with the burglar's next telephone call, which was expected at any moment. I explained to them the importance of obtaining the longest sample possible, for the reasons just outlined above, and they duly passed on this advice to the old lady. When I received the tape-recorded copy of the burglar's next call to her I was really quite astonished at the extent to which she had been able to take control of the conversation and get a substantial sample.

The burglar opened the dialogue in the rough, bullying tones typical of such situations, and the old lady, let us call her Mrs A, answered, in a deceptively meek style, his questions about her willingness to pay the money, and to co-operate by not involving the police. She managed to satisfy him on those matters, and he then moved on to the details of how Mrs A was to make the money available to him. Here Mrs A began to exert control. When he was only part way through the directions she asked him to stop for a moment and let her get something to write on. He paused while she did this, but when she announced her return and he was about to continue from where he had left off, she claimed that she had forgotten what he had already said, and would he please go over it again because she was an old lady whose memory didn't always work very well. He started from the beginning again, but he had not got very far when she asked him to stop once more. This time she told him that she had a heart condition, and that all this excitement had tired her. Would he please hold on for a moment while she got herself a glass of water and a chair to sit on? This procedure continued, with variations, for some considerable time, with Mrs A gradually persuading the burglar, by her apparent weakness and willingness to co-operate, to repeat his instructions a number of times. Towards the end the burglar had dropped his hectoring manner and was becoming quite felicitous towards Mrs A - was she sure she was able to continue? Was she sure everything was clear, or should he go over the instructions again? And so on, and so on!

The whole conversation was recorded, and when I compared the now extensive sample of the burglar with that of a suspect I found very close similarities between them. On the basis of that and other evidence a man was eventually charged and found guilty of the burglary and of attempting to extort money from Mrs A. From the latter's point of view everything ended happily, as happily as it could under the circumstances that is, in that her painting was discovered to be undamaged. In due course, i.e. after the court hearing in which it was produced in evidence, it was returned to her.

This is the best example in all the cases I have worked on of a victim exerting control over the would-be extortionist, though not the only one. It is unusual, I think, in that it features a member of the public, Mrs A, with , as far as I ever discovered, no training in such techniques, but who took to them, so to speak, as a duck takes to water.

I am sure it is not unknown in other walks of forensic life for criminals to discover that their prospective victim is more than a match for them. When the victim is decidedly not equal to the psychological onslaught of, say, a persistent anonymous telephone caller however, the sample which arises is, in contradiction to the principle I expressed above of 'maximal sample', too long for all of it to be of use. Here the phonetician must select those passages which contain, in the most compact way, those features of pronunciation he has observed to be typical of the subject in the rest of the sample.

The most extreme example I have ever heard of in this context was the case of a woman who was persecuted by anonymous telephone callers, usually a husband and wife partnership, but occasionally involving other callers obviously known to them. The content of the calls was, with very occasional exceptions, of an almost unbelievable level of obscenity. The recipient of the calls, let us call her Mrs R, had been receiving them over a considerable period of time. A typical call would start like this:

Mrs R: 'Hello.'
Mrs X: 'Don't know why you put the phone down for, love?'
Mrs R: 'I didn't put the phone down, that's you.'
Mrs X: 'No, it was you, love.'
Mrs R: 'No.'
Mrs X: 'Can't hear you, love.'
Mrs R: 'You're really sick.'
Mrs X: 'What'd you say, love?'
Mrs R: 'I said you're really sick.'
Mrs X: 'Don't be silly, love.'
Mrs R: 'No, I'm not being silly.'
Mrs X: 'You're the one that's sick, love.'
Mrs R: 'No.'
Mrs X: 'You are, love.'
Mrs R: 'No.'

and so on, and so on!

A typical conclusion would be along these lines, picking up the conversation towards the end:

Mrs R: 'Do what?'
Mrs X: 'You heard, love.'
Mrs R: 'No, I didn't.'
Mrs X: 'Not right for the other children mixing with them, love.'
Mrs R: 'My children mixing with other children?'
Mrs X: 'Mm, they got fleas love, haven't they?'
Mrs R: 'Oh, leave it out!'
Mrs X: 'They have, love, they're undernourished.'
Mrs R: 'No.'
Mrs X: 'Go to the vet's, love.'
Mrs R: 'No.'
Mrs X: (inaudible)
Mrs R: 'Pardon.'
Mrs X: 'You heard, love.'
Mrs R: 'Did I?'
Mrs X: 'Go on, have yourself a scrub round the crutch-piece, love.'
Mrs R: 'You're sick, you're really sick. Ain't you got any . . .'
       (receiver replaced by Mrs X)

It is difficult to imagine ourselves in the position of Mrs R, but if we try to do so, our first reaction is surely going to be something along the lines of 'I can't stand this, I'm going to hang up', and then to do just that. Indeed, there were frequent occasions when Mrs R said, in so many words 'I can't stand this', and others when she said that the callers made her feel sick (and there were certainly times in listening to the tapes when I shared that feeling!), but, quite incredibly, she does not terminate the conversation. In fact she never terminated the conversation, no matter how strongly she objected to what the caller was saying. It would be possible to understand her reaction of shocked inertia if the calls were infrequent, or one-off, where she would have had no chance of adjusting to what was happening by evolving a defensive strategy. Such inertia is quite common when ordinary people are subjected to pressures over the telephone which they are unable to cope with because they are totally unfamiliar. I have noticed this on many occasions, including a very unpleasant kidnap case, where the distressed father of the child received the call telling him where to leave the money, and giving him a list of the unpleasant things that would happen to his son if anything went wrong. When the kidnapper had finished his business, conducted in a most brutal manner, he ended the conversation by saying 'Good-bye', whereupon the father responded with a conventionally polite 'Good-bye' of his own. Clearly, the father was distraught, and reacted without thinking, and this, as I have said above, is the usual way in which people do react in such circumstances. However, that was hardly the situation with Mrs R, the transcripts of the conversations I heard, and these were not in fact the first of them, amounted to a staggering 300 pages! She had built up, potentially at any rate, an enormous body of experience in handling the calls, and yet she never once, in dozens of allegedly sickening conversations, put down the receiver before the caller did! During the progress of the 300 pages of transcript it is not possible to discern the slightest advance in Mrs R's control techniques – her reactions to the caller are precisely the same in the last of the conversations as they were in the first of them, and it therefore makes no difference whereabouts in the transcripts one selects the sample text from. For example, there are many occasions when the caller, whether the male or female, leads Mrs R into asking a question, and then hangs up without answering it, the precise opposite of what should be happening if Mrs R intended to control things, as exemplified in the following extract:

Mr X: ' . . . the old woman told me you was asking about me.'
Mrs R: 'Oh, I don't ask about you, you're sick.'
Mr X: 'I'm not sick, love.'
Mrs R: 'I think so.'
Mr X: 'No I'm not, love.'
Mrs R: 'So what do you want?' (Receiver replaced by Mr X!).

She appears almost mesmerised by the callers, afraid to take the initiative against her persecutors. Yet, in fact, some initiative must have been taken by somebody, because the matter was placed in the hands of the police; otherwise the calls would not have been recorded, of course. Added to the sickening obscenity of the husband/wife team was their stupidity and arrogance, in that it appeared that all the calls were made on their own telephone at their home! It seems likely, knowing as they did the control they were able to exert over Mrs R, that they really believed she would not make an official complaint against them. They were mistaken in that, it seems, and yet one cannot but wonder whether the husband's claim made in the calls he originated, that she secretly enjoyed his conversation, did not represent an insightful psychological observation on his part. The fact that he was a person of the greatest crudity on other levels would not, I think, rule out the possibility of such sensitivity in this particular direction. The following extract is typical of the kind of conversation Mr X originated:

Mrs R: 'Hello.'
Mr X: 'Hello, love.'
Mrs R: 'What do you want?'
Mr X: 'I thought I'd give you a ring.'
Mrs R: 'Really? What for?'
Mr X: 'Well, you like me talking to you, don't you?'
Mrs R: 'Oh, leave it out. You're sick.'
Mr X: 'Don't say fucking "Leave it out, you're sick". You like it.'

(picking up on the third transcript page of this conversation)

Mr X: 'How's your old arsehole?'
Mrs R: 'You're filth.'
Mr X: 'I'm not filth, love.'
Mrs R: 'Yeah.'

Mr X: 'For fuck's sake, she keeps saying I'm filth. I love your arsehole, the other day in that queue with them leather trousers on.'

Mrs R: 'I never had the leather trousers on the other day.'

The conversation continues in similar vein for another three pages of transcript, and ends typically enough with a question from Mrs R: 'What interest is it . . .?' She never completes her question, because Mr X hangs up in the middle of it!

The suspects, husband and wife, were interviewed separately by the police. The husband chatted quite confidently, arguing that, since nobody in their right mind would make obscene calls on their own domestic telephone as they could so easily be traced, it stood to reason that he had not made the calls in question! The sample of his speech was very good, since it was both long and clearly recorded. It displayed the same characteristics as I had already noted in the case of the unknown male caller. These were, in particular, an unusual, rather hoarse kind of voice quality, and a slightly breathless effect achieved by his habit of whispering or skipping very quickly over unstressed syllables. For example, he produced no voicing in the italic part of the phrase: 'I *could have* kept on making them', and truncated the syllable 'out' in the phrase: 'come with*out* me glasses' to such a degree that the transcript writer simply did not perceive it, and wrote the precise opposite of what the suspect actually said. This 'tripping' manner of speaking is, I believe, usually to be found in young girls, and to meet it in such a person as this particular suspect is, surely, the very height of incongruity! As a result of these similarities I was able to report my conviction that he and the male X were one and the same. He had apparently boundless confidence in his own invulnerability, a confidence which, as it eventually transpired, was shaken.

His wife, when she came to be interviewed, was an entirely different proposition, having clearly resolved not to co-operate in providing a sample of her speech. For one thing, the unknown female caller had been responsible for the great majority of the recorded calls, and for another, had tried sporadically to conceal her own accent by adopting an accent which was so random and outlandish that it approached the bizarre. It was very obviously a counterfeit accent, and there was in the recorded samples a vast body of material in which her basic accent showed through, remembering that there were 300 pages of transcript. If the female suspect had made the Mrs X calls, she would not wish to permit any comparison of the two samples. Throughout the interview she refused to answer any questions, beyond giving her name, address and telephone number. Otherwise she said words to the effect: 'I'm not answering it on my solicitor's advice'. It is, of course, a suspect's legal right to remain silent. The resulting sample was far too short for any high-level positive identification, and little could be said beyond the fact that, in so far as her speech could be compared with that of the unknown female, there seemed to be similarities and no obvious differences, and that they *could*, therefore, be the same.

As it transpired, these identifications could not be tested in court, because the prosecution failed to get the papers entered within the statutory period of six months allowed for the purpose. The case was, therefore, 'out of time', which meant that all proceedings had to be dropped and the suspects informed that no further action would be taken against them in this case. Nobody, then, was charged with or tried for the offences, and no connection can be made, in legal terms, between Mr and Mrs X and the suspects. The fact that Mrs R received no further obscene telephone calls after the investigation is, perhaps, entirely coincidental. I have been involved in a number of 'out of time' cases, and I always experience the same disappointment that my work, together with that of quite a large number of others, is apparently wasted. Despite the dire threats uttered by senior police officers of heads being caused to roll, such cases do occur with more than desirable frequency, from their point of view, but at least in the present instance there seems to have been a not entirely negative outcome.

If the speech samples are not rejected by the phonetician either on the grounds of their lack of clarity or because the text is inadequate, or both, of course, the next operation would be that of screening for obvious phonetic discrepancies. In practice, this would normally overlap to some extent with the preceeding checks, although they are, obviously, quite different kinds of activity. At this stage of the procedings I would be listening to the voice quality, voice pitch characteristics and segmental features of pronunciation (Chapter 2). Unless there is some suggestion that at least one of the speakers might be attempting to disguise his accent, any major discrepancies at this point would probably lead to the opinion that the speakers are different people.

It would, perhaps, be helpful here to discuss the various ways in which speech samples might be found to be different. As stated earlier (Chapter 2), voice quality, voice pitch and speech rhythm are customarily placed under the single heading: suprasegmental features. Differences in all of the items under this heading would almost certainly be interpreted as evidence that the samples were spoken by different people; apparently parallel similarities would not, however, indicate that the speakers are the same, only that they *could* be. There is, therefore, a skewing of evidential weight in favour of the negative indications, and it is not possible to suggest that two speakers must be the same on the basis of similarities in this area; one would always be looking for confirmatory evidence from the segmental pronunciation, i.e. that of vowels and consonants.

One of the implications of this principle is that phoneticians are, almost universally, disinclined to deal with speech samples in languages of which they do not have a very good knowledge. Along with other phoneticians I am constantly being asked to carry out comparisons, for example, of samples which are all in a language which I do not know, such as Arabic or Punjabi, or where one sample is in English and the other(s) in another, to me unknown language. Any comparisons would have to be based solely on supra-segmental features, and these reveal themselves to be unreliable in terms of establishing any high-level positive identification. The most one could expect is a *possible* identification. Comparison of the speaker's segmental phonetic features is not possible, because one must have an idea of what the target pronunciation is in any given instance; one needs to know the system. For example, it would be possible to find two identical vowel qualities in two English samples, but these would not contribute to a positive identification, because one was from a northern speaker saying 'back' whilst the other was from a London speaker saying 'buck'. Comparable problems occur in all languages, of course, and it clearly needs a good knowledge of any particular language to allow for them, and to compare like with like. When I am approached on this matter, my first reaction is to explain why it is not possible to compare samples in a language one does not know, and then to try to recommend a phonetician who does know the language. That is extremely difficult, not to say impossible, in the case of, for example, any of the languages of the Indian sub-continent. Under extreme pressure, because no such phonetician has been found or has been forthcoming, I have agreed occasionally to given an opinion, but I have always made clear the considerable limitations of that opinion.

When looking for discrepancies in vowels and consonants, one must begin with a comparison of systems, for the reasons outlined above. Differences of a systemic character between samples would be a strong indication that they were produced by different speakers, although this could be complicated by the phenomenon of 'accent switching' (Chapter 5). The conditions under which such a complication might occur are fairly clear, and do not apply to the vast majority of cases. Differences in vowel systems of an obvious kind would be the presence or absence of the RP vowel in 'much'. Many non-RP speakers do not have this vowel in their system at all, and one possibility is that they could produce 'much' with the same vowel as RP 'look'. There are further possibilities, too, but the point is that the systems are different if that vowel is present in one, but not in the other. A less obvious difference, at least to RP-speakers, though not necessarily to others, is the maintaining of a distinction between the pronunciations of words like 'side' and 'sighed', as is done in many Scottish accents.

Having discovered discrepancies in neither the supra-segmental features nor the phonemic system, the phonetician's final task is to compare the detailed realisations of those phonemes. Even when all the other features are found to coincide, it is still common for differences to emerge on this level of analysis. At this point it is necessary for the phonetician to decide whether these differences are within the normal allophonic range for the accent in question, and, consequently, that the speakers are, on whatever level of probability, the same person, or whether those differences are more likely to indicate that the samples were spoken by different people. The reader will, I hope, recall the discussion of speech-variability in the Introduction, which is highly relevant here, and also that concerning the status of instrumental analysis. In making his decision one way or the other, the phonetician must exercise his judgment on the basis of his experience. (All forensic phoneticians have encountered samples in which they simply could not arrive at such a decision; when that happens, the third option is taken, i.e. to report that they find the samples to be on the borderline of their positive/negative categories, and to refrain from offering an opinion.) Recourse to spectrographic and/or other analysis in this problematic kind of case is not likely to help in that decision-making process, because it will inevitably introduce its own complications in the matter of interpretation.

This discussion brings us to the end of Chapter 4, in which various aspects of forensic phonetics have been considered. The following presentation of cases should help to illustrate some of the matters dealt with in all the preceeding chapters.

Chapter 5

Cases

I have selected for inclusion here those of my cases which, I believe, will be of some interest to the general reader as well as to the specialist. I have also chosen those cases in which I felt I learnt something of value - they will not necessarily be 'victorious' cases, therefore. It would have been logical, too, to begin with the first forensic case that I was involved in. As it fortunately transpires, that case was one of particular, and formative significance, and I shall, then, do the obvious thing and begin at the beginning.

The background to the case is that in the 1960s there was an intensive campaign by the police in London against the underworld 'empire' of the notorious Kray twins, Ronnie and Reggie. As part of this campaign, a dragnet was put out with the intention of bringing into the light of day any and all of the friends and associates of the Krays. There was, in consequence, the highest level of police activity that the criminal world, or anyone else for that matter, had seen for many years in London. Even the most distant contact of the Krays was likely to be brought in for questioning.

That period was, clearly, not exactly the best time for a foreigner of criminal tendencies to choose to visit London, but that is precisely when the subject of the case, let us identify him by the initial J, elected to do so. As the details of J's visit to London unfold, it will become progressively more obvious that J, at that time at least, was on a run of bad luck, evidenced by a series of wrong decisions on his part.

Wrong decision number one, then, was to come to London in the first place. Wrong decision number two was to make contact with members of the underworld, and to try to interest them in certain forged bonds which J was handling. Given their awareness of the general police presence on the underworld as a whole, they were understandably reluctant to get involved with J's operation. The latter was clearly very frustrated at his lack of progress in an undertaking which, to him at least, looked both fairly free of danger and, potentially, highly rewarding financially. However, instead of accepting that the prospects of any success were too dim, cutting his losses and heading for home, J decided to remain in London and struggle on. This was wrong decision number three.

Driven by desperation, he racked his brains for some means of getting things moving. Unfortunately for him, he came up with what he saw as the bright idea of mentioning his connection with the Krays to certain people in a number of London underworld locations. He had hopes that by doing so he would open doors hitherto closed to him. He was certainly right in that respect, but hardly in ways he could have envisaged! Had he been gifted with foresight enough to see the outcome of this decision, he would certainly have left for home there and then.

This last decision of J's had far-reaching consequences and was, arguably, something of a major accomplishment in the art of self-destruction; as we shall see in due course, it was in fact mistaken on two vital matters. Firstly, as wrong decision number four, it had the initial and deceptive appearance of success, in that it did indeed secure J's admittance to the presence of an associate of the Krays. This man, let us call him X, had had to go into hospital for an operation of a fairly minor character, and, in order to secure the privacy of his own room, had entered one of the private hospitals in Harley Street. J happily went along to his meeting with X, and talked with him for about half an hour on matters of general interest, before embarking on the sales promotion for his own project. J described his acquaintance with the Krays, as well as his own business background in the United States – he was, it seemed, owner of a 1 per cent share in a pop-star of the time, one whose precipitous rise to stardom was followed in very short order by his equally, if not even more precipitous fall. J had a number of other, legitimate business interests, too, but these were all of a similarly unrewarding nature from the financial point of view. J did not receive from these various undertakings what he regarded as an adequate income for the kind of life that he would have liked to be able to set up for himself. It was for this reason that he had devised the project of the counterfeit bonds. He had believed that he would have more success in making an advantageous deal in London, and in any case, as he said, was glad of the change of scenery. After a slow start in negotiations, which he now perceived as having been put safely behind him, J was anxious to make up for lost time. He was, therefore, particularly keen on discussing with X the most expeditious arrangements that could be made for the handling of the forged bonds, which he had taken the initiative of bringing with him from the USA. His bed-bound contact showed a good deal of enthusiasm for the project, and J was clearly delighted at this, because it was the first positive reaction he had encountered since arriving in London some weeks before. He was, therefore, inclined to take this as encouragement, and spoke in a very relaxed and open way about his plans.

His listener seemed to go along with all of J's suggestions, but what he omitted to tell J at any point during the interview was that the room was bugged, and that the whole of their conversation was being recorded by the police! Some time ago, in return for their acceptance of a plea by him to a relatively minor criminal offence, X had agreed with the police to turn 'Queen's evidence', and to co-operate in securing the arrest of as many of his former colleagues in the underworld as he reasonably could. Using as a cover the occasion of his genuine need to undergo an operation, the police had arranged with X, and with the authorities of the hospital which he had agreed to enter for the operation, to set up a concealed recording device in X's room. X had been instructed to invite any member of the Kray circle to visit him in this room, and to engage them in conversations which could prove to be incriminating and possibly lead to their arrest. Having claimed to be an associate of the Krays, J came into that category. He had been permitted to enter this trap, and had duly incriminated himself in a most enthusiastic manner. The police had a substantial recorded sample of J's speech, together with details of a crime of which they might conceivably never have heard, or possibly heard about too late to catch J after the bonds had been negotiated.

Falling into the trap was bad enough, even by J's standards, but the error was greatly compounded when it emerged that J really should not have been admitted to the trap at all. When he claimed that he knew the Krays, he was, in fact, taking certain liberties with the truth. (Wrong decision number five.) That he knew *of* the Krays was certainly true, but at that time everybody knew of the Krays, including the most unlikely people. At the very most, J can only have seen them from across the room in some public place, and it was virtually certain that he had never actually spoken with them. J had built upon this tenuous connection in his desperation to advance his project. This was another mistake, the implications of which only became clear, and painfully so, to J some time later.

The immediate result of J's visit to X in the private hospital was, as one might have expected, that J was arrested, and charged with importing and handling forged bonds. When confronted with the evidence of the tape-recording of his alleged conversation with X, J listened to the speakers' voices a number of times. He then announced to his solicitor that the person alleged to be him on the tape was, in fact, someone else. He instructed his solicitor to find a 'voice-print' expert, who would soon be able to demonstrate J's innocence to the court. With the help of the Law Society, J's solicitor got into contact with a colleague of mine who was, and indeed still is, a specialist in experimental and instrumental phonetics, acoustic phonetics, in fact. The latter's first task was to explain to the solicitor, and in terms very much as to be found in Chapter 3 of this book, why there was no such thing as a voice-print. He further explained what kinds of help the phonetician would be in a position to offer, i.e. instrumental examination of the tape itself, and auditory analysis and comparison of the two speech samples: J and the alleged J. After conferring with J his solicitor opted for auditory analysis and comparison. My colleague said that he would feel happier if he were able to bring into the case two new members of the department who were auditory phoneticians, although both unpractised in forensic work. J agreed, and so I found myself, together with my two colleagues, making for Brixton Prison in order to interview and record J's speech.

J had been remanded in custody in that prison because there was very little prospect of his being able to raise bail to an adequate level. Had he been bailed in any case, it seemed rather more than an even chance that he would seize the opportunity to disappear across the Atlantic, and to be seen no more in London. The police, therefore, strongly resisted bail, and J was consequently confined to Brixton Prison to await trial. Most people locked up under such circumstances agree that it is some way from being the best time of their lives. In J's case, though, there were special and unusual circumstances which made his sojourn there rather more than usually disagreeable. When J had, quite untruthfully, used the name and reputation of the Krays to secure his own illegal ends, this had not passed unnoticed in their circles. It was a by no means unreasonable reaction on the part of their associates to take exception to the fact that J had tried to exploit them. This was something to which they were not accustomed, nor did they intend to allow any possible development of such a practice into a habit. Thus, when J found himself in prison he simultaneously found himself enclosed in uncomfortable proximity to friends of the Krays. He was threatened, verbally abused and physically attacked, and sustained a number of injuries. J requested that he be put in solitary confinement for his own safety. Such confinement is, basically, intended as a punishment for offenders against the prison rules and regulations, and is, in consequence, neither pleasant nor popular. Prisoners would not normally expect to spend more than days, or at most weeks there, but J was no ordinary prisoner, and his problems of no ordinary measure. His case dragged on and on, through one legal complication after another, and, by the time he actually came to trial, J had spent the best part of a year in solitary confinement.

When my colleagues and I recorded him, he had already been in solitary confinement for many months. He spoke with us for about half an hour, during which time he claimed that the alleged J was definitely not him, because he sounded different and because he used expressions which the real J would never use, and so on. The recording quality was good, especially considering the unpromising acoustic environment.

That was my first visit to a prison, and, despite many subsequent visits to Brixton and other prisons to record speech samples, I have never got used to the disquieting and uncomfortable atmosphere to be met in them.

Together with my auditory phonetician colleague, I listened to the two samples: the real and the alleged J. Both samples were of comparable length and content, i.e. fully adequate for our purposes. The clarity of the real J sample was very good, but that of the alleged J less so. There were many clicks and bangs of an electronic character, due to the recording technique, to which I shall return in a moment. Despite that, the alleged J sample afforded us ample material which was clear enough for phonetic analysis.

We had been given to understand that J came from New York, and so we expected to find some features of such an accent in

J's speech. However, upon examination of his sample we could
find no features which deviated from General American: he was
fully rhotic, i.e. he used 'r' in all positions in the word. A typical
New York accent would be non-rhotic, with 'r' only before
vowels, or, possibly, semi-rhotic, with 'r' before consonants and
pauses only when the mid central vowel in, for example, 'first'
was involved. In the matter of his other consonantal features, he
produced 'th' sounds (i.e. dental fricatives) correctly, that is, as
expected in General American, as well as other features. With
respect to his vowel system, the same was true: typical New
York features were conspicuously absent. For example, in a
word like 'long' he produced a pure, back, open unrounded
vowel, and not a diphthongal form which would be expected of
a New York accent. This absence of a New York accent in J's
speech led us to conclude either that J probably did not come
from New York, or that he was from a social group which did
not speak with a local accent, or that he had modified his
pronunciation at some time.

In any event, our next task was to discover whether the
alleged J spoke with the same, or a similar accent. We checked
out all the accent features that we had observed in the J sample,
and found that in every respect the accent of the alleged J was
the same as the admitted J. This in itself was a positive identification, but not on a very high level because the General
American accent, of course, is spoken by a considerable number
of people. Even taking into account the very closely similar
voice qualities and pitch features of the alleged and the admitted J, one would still be dealing with possibilities.

We believed the deciding factor in establishing a positive identification would be the coincidence of the details of the realisations of the abstract units, the variants of the phonemes
themselves that is, in the two samples. We therefore compared
the phonetic characteristics of, particularly, the vowels, in order
to confirm that the same degree of, for example, openness,
backness, roundedness and so on, was present in both samples.
No matter what segmental detail we checked, the answer was
always the same: we could find no differences between the
speech of the alleged and the admitted J which did not fall
within our understanding of the normal allophonic range for his
accent.

There were some differences between the samples in the
voice pitch characteristics, i.e. in the average pitch and

intonation. Although our observations were entirely auditory, and based on direct comparisons of the two samples, we had found that the difference between the average pitch level of the alleged J sample and that of the admitted J was of a substantial order, and that the average pitch of the admitted J was lower. Interestingly though, examination of the intonation in the form of the excursions of pitch to very high and/or very low, or extra high and/or extra low, revealed that such excursions were relatively rare in the alleged J sample, but quite common in the admitted J sample. Given the weight of the segmental and voice quality similarities mentioned above, we felt it was very unlikely that these pitch differences could be indications that the alleged and the admitted J were, in fact, different people. It seemed to us far more probable that these differences were due to the different mental and physical states of the same speaker in quite different situations. The alleged J was, it will be recalled, speaking freely and enthusiastically with a sympathetic audience. The pitch features here are appropriate to a speaker who feels both lively and relaxed. In the case of the admitted J, however, that is far from being the case. At the time the sample was taken, J had been in solitary confinement for many months, with few opportunities to converse in any extended way. He was also, if only in his own imagination, under constant threat of physical violence. As a result of these pressures, J must have been depressed, and at the same time, far from relaxed. Further elements contributing to his psychological condition on that occasion were that he was giving an interview to three people he had not met before, that they were recording it, and that the outcome of their examination of his speech could, potentially, prove crucial in the advantageous progress of his case. We believed that these factors explained the pitch differences in a feasible way. Our final conclusion, then, was that the alleged and the admitted J were, in fact, the same person, and that we felt no doubt that that was the case.

We made our opinion known to J's solicitor, who took this setback with professional aplomb. He in turn reported it to J. Having considered the problem for some time, J came to the conclusion that, yes, it must have been him all the time on the police recording, but that he did not recognise himself because the police had edited and re-ordered his utterances. They had arranged them in such a way that he had been made to appear to incriminate himself, whereas, of course, his conversation had been of a totally innocent and honest character. He therefore took the second option that my colleague had offered him at the very beginning of the case: an instrumental examination of the tape.

I mentioned earlier that the alleged J sample was rather noisy, with frequent electronic clicks and bangs, and with other interference. This was the result of the recording set-up itself. At that time the police did not command the most advanced technology, and in any case, the technology of surreptitious recording was not very advanced. The microphone was located in the telephone, and the whole system had to be plugged into the mains supply. This meant that any activity on the mains, in the form of switching on or off, etc., came over on the tape as a noise. Having examined the tape, my colleague came to the conclusion that there was so much extraneous noise on it, and of such a character that he believed that any amount of editing could have been carried out, and that any traces of it could have been concealed in the general noise events. It looked, at last, as if something was going right for J.

My colleague reported his opinion to J's solicitor, and he, in his turn reported both to J and to the prosecution. Perhaps surprisingly, the latter did not contest that opinion, or have it tested by their own expert. Instead, they simply accepted it, and agreed to drop that particular item from their evidence. It will be noted that J's solicitor had not previously reported the positive identification which my other colleague and I had made. Not only was he legally entitled to supress information potentially detrimental to his client's interests, but he would have been, and still would be guilty of failing properly to represent his client. I have known several instances in which solicitors have withdrawn from cases, having refused to enter a pleas of 'not guilty' for their clients when they have been given reason to believe that they were probably guilty. That did not happen in this case.

Having spent a whole year on remand, not only in custody, but in solitary confinement, J must certainly have been relieved when he was eventually brought to trial. He was found guilty of handling forged bonds, and was sentenced to thirteen months imprisonment, and to deportation to the USA when he had served his sentence. Having already spent a year in prison, J had only one more month to do, and then he would be returned to the bosom of his native land, and without further expenditure on his part.

For once in J's affairs everything went as planned, perhaps because he was not responsible for planning them, and he was duly deported. By this time he would probably not have been in the least surprised if he had been involved in a motor accident on the way to the airport, or if the plane had crashed. However, neither these nor any other mishaps befell J in London, and he disappeared gratefully from our sight. From time to time over the years my thoughts have returned to J. I have wondered whether his experiences in London proved to be traumatic, and to have acted as an aversion therapy in relation to crime; he was so obviously a failure as a criminal. I hope very much that he has become a successful and legitimate businessman in his own country, but have considerable doubt that he would ever have made a return trip to London.

I remember this case particularly well, partly because it was my first, but also because it opened my eyes to some character-istics of our legal system of which I had not previously been aware. I have already mentioned one: the legal right of the defence side to conceal information potentially against their client's interests. As the result of recent legislation, defence can no longer spring surprise witnesses and evidence on the prosecu-tion, but it has not affected their right to supress potential evidence which is not of advantage to their client. In the past, defence had been permitted to do both, whereas the prosecution have always been obliged to serve details of their case on the defence, and at an adequate interval before the trial to allow the preparation of a viable defence case. This imbalance originates, as I understand it, in the very laudable desire to give the defen-dant every possible resource against the prosecution, who could, after all, mobilise all the forces of the legal system against him. The result of this situation for the expert witness is that, although having been consulted by the prosecution, he often arrives at conclusions not advantageous to the prosecution case. Following the passing over of his views to the other side, he finds himself acting for the defence. On the other hand, if he is consulted by the defence, and arrives at an opinion not favour-able to them, the results of his work are quietly disposed of, and nothing more is heard of it. I have long believed that this problem of maintaining a fair balance between the power of the legal system as set against the individual, arises solely from our adversarial system, which is also accusatorial in the sense that it divides legal practice in the criminal area into sides set one against the other. It became clear to me in the case of J, and nothing I have experienced subsequently in nearly 300 cases has changed that understanding, that the objective of many criminal cases is not primarily to see justice done, but to see your side win.

After the J case I was not consulted by any defence solicitor for more than a year. My first thought was, naturally, that it was purely coincidental; however, when I mentioned the dearth of defence cases in a casual conversation with a civilian employee of the police, his immediate response was sadly representative of the attitudes prevalent within the adversary system. His claim was that I had not been consulted by defence solicitors because my colleague and I had come to an independent conclusion, and one not to their liking since it was against their case. Defence solicitors, he alleged, are only interested in consulting 'experts' who can be relied upon to produce evidence in favour of their clients. His suggestion was that there are certain 'experts' known to the legal profession who are prepared to doctor their opinions to suit the requirements of whichever side happens to consult them. I believe that both his allegations are true: there are such solicitors and there are such 'experts'. However, I would not wish to give the impression to the reader that I feel such people are at all numerous. I would certainly not want to generalise to the extent that my police colleague did, but whether he was right or not, his attitude is a typical product of the system.

In another case a few years later, heard in Bristol Crown Court, I was acting for the prosecution. My evidence related to a very brief hoax telephone call to the police which had been recorded, and which constituted my X sample. There was another, control sample which was adequate in all respects for phonetic analysis and comparison. The two samples showed many similarities, but two slight differences in the vowel qualities. Because of this, and the relative brevity of the X sample. I had only been prepared to say that the two samples *could* have been spoken by the same person. I had mentioned both the vowel discrepancies and the less than ideal length of one of the samples. In giving my evidence, both in chief and under cross-examination, I made these points clear. Afterwards, as I was leaving the court, a police employee criticised my evidence, because, as he said, he had not been able to tell whether I was on the side of the prosecution or the defence. I tried to explain that the expert witness is not on any side, but says what he has found irrespective of which side consulted him. I am by no means convinced that he accepted my explanation. Even if he did, his first observation was an honest statement of his expectations of an expert 'on his side'. It is greatly to be regretted that such attitudes are prevalent, but, as I said above, I believe them to arise inevitably from our system – some people will always be more concerned about winning than about hearing the experts' expressions of doubt in their own conclusions, whatever the system, but ours encourages, and indeed substantially rewards the winners. I shall return to a discussion of this fundamental problem in Chapter 6 – The Future, where I shall look at some implications of the points raised here.

The next case I would like to describe was one set in Northern Ireland. Inevitably, it took place against the background of terrorism still so unhappily endemic there, although the participants themselves were not members of any terrorist organisation such as the IRA, and so on. The case was also of particular interest to me because it was the first in which 'accent-switching' was involved to my certain knowledge. It will make subsequent matters clearer if I discuss this phenomenon at this point, rather than deferring it. I shall return to the case itself in due course.

Accent-switching refers to the changes made by a given speaker in his accent for purposes other than those of deception. It must, therefore, be clearly distinguished from the adoption of a counterfeit accent (see Chapter 4) by a would-be deceiver. In the latter case, the adopted accent is not 'real' to the speaker, but is chosen by him as a potentially good means of covering up his own accent, which is, of course, 'real'. Since the accent used in deception is not part of the speaker's normal behaviour, he is likely to be unsuccessful in that attempt, even if he chooses an accent with which he is familiar for other reasons.

In the case of the accent-switcher, however, both accents are equally real. He switches from one to the other, for reasons to be discussed below, often quite unconsciously, whereas the deceiver switches consciously on all occasions. When a person switches accent, it is done, by definition, successfully, because he achieves the effect which, consciously or otherwise, he has set out to produce.

Accent-switching almost always has a sociological/psychological explanation, and is best understood if we look at some typical contexts in which it is known to occur. The English reader needs to be given such examples, because accent-switching is not usually a part of English socio-linguistic practice. In most countries there is a marked difference between the standard form of speech and the regional form, and this difference is very often found on all relevant levels of language: vocabulary, syntax, morphology, phonology and phonetics. Even if this difference is evinced on only one level, e.g. phonetics, speakers in other societies feel the need to switch their accents when they are moving from a non-regional environment such as their place of work where they are professionals in the company of other professionals, to their home-town, where they are amongst their families and friends. This is certainly the case with professional people in Germany, Japan and so on. They say that their behaviour would be interpreted as distinctly unfriendly if they failed to revert to their regional accents in such contexts. The English situation is usually quite different, though, because for us accents are associated with class rather than region. An Englishman who has moved from the working class to the professional class, and who has changed his accent in the process, is not likely to be well-received by his erstwhile associates who know that he has changed his accent if he reverts to his regional form with them, but uses a different accent with other, professional people. They would quite possibly feel that he was mocking or patronising them. Where accent is not socially based, i.e. in most of the rest of the world, such embarrassment is unusual, if not, indeed, unknown.

Accent-switching can be carried out for reasons other than those just mentioned. For example, a speaker can switch accent in order to distance himself from the people he is talking with; he can switch to exclude an outsider, and he can switch to make himself intelligible to an outsider, or to bring the outsider into the circle. A number of the reasons given here for accent-switching occur in the Northern Ireland case, and I therefore think it appropriate to return to that case.

A prosperous farming family, let us call them Radley, received a number of telephone calls from at least one unknown male claiming to represent the Ulster Volunteer Force, which is a proscribed, Protestant paramilitary organisation in Northern Ireland. The caller(s) demanded money from the Radleys, against the threat that random members of their family would be shot if the money were not paid. Such is the situation in

Northern Ireland that if someone threatens to kill someone else, it is taken seriously, at its face value. In other parts of the British Isles such a threat would probably be treated as a joke, in the first instance at any rate; not a particularly amusing joke, to be sure, but not meant seriously, nevertheless. In Northern Ireland, though, such an utterance is not usually intended as a joke, particularly when it is issued by people claiming to be representatives of the UVF against a Roman Catholic family. The Radleys were extremely distraught at these telephone messages, and, as ordinary and sensible people, contacted the Royal Ulster Constabulary. The RUC promptly put a recording device on the Radley's telephone, and waited for the next call. This was not long in coming, and in fact four extensive calls were recorded over the next few days, all from the same caller(s) the family had heard before, and all to the same effect: the Radleys must pay protection money to the UVF or face arbitrary assassination. They agreed to go along with some kind of payment, but before any meetings could be arranged, events took a different course.

Some members of the family happened to have called in at their local police station, and while they were waiting there they heard a voice they thought they recognised. From the other side of a partition in the police station came what sounded to them like the voice of the young man that they had previously heard as the (principal) maker of the putative UVF calls. Naturally enough, they could hardly believe their ears, but told the police about the reaction which all of them had had to the voice of the unseen speaker. The RUC responded by holding the young man for questioning.

The suspect, let us call him M, had been in the police station on a matter which bore no relationship to the affairs of the Radleys. His interview by the RUC did not raise that issue, but concentrated on other aspects of M's dealings with the law. The interview was recorded, and a copy of it brought to me so that I could compare the voice of M with the voice(s) of the unknown caller(s) to the Radleys.

I first listened to the X calls, and felt able to conclude that all four had in all probability been spoken by the same individual. Despite the presence of discrepancies, particularly in one of the calls, I was satisfied that such discrepancies fell within the range of normal variation in that accent. All the samples were produced with a variety of Northern Irish English which is usually referred to as Scots Irish. Some salient features of this, which distinguish it from Irish Irish, are the widespread use of the glottal stop, even to reinforce voiced consonants as in 'Radley', as opposed to its non-occurrence; the use of a back rounded diphthong in words like 'cold', 'go', etc., as opposed to the Irish Irish front rounded diphthong; the correct pronunciation of dental fricatives, as opposed to their realisation as dental stops, and so on.

When I listened to the sample of M's speech, and compared it with X, I found both similarities and differences. The first were in the general accent features appropriate to Northern Ireland, and in the voice quality and voice pitch features, whilst the second lay in all those features I have alluded to above which typically distinguish the Scots Irish speaker from the Irish Irish speaker. I was aware of the possibility of accent-switching in the Northern Ireland community. It is, it seems, very common there, but no matter how common it may be, it is never possible to say with certainty that it has occurred in any given sample, unless the speaker switches during the recording. In the present instance there was no sign that it had happened. The phonetician must, as any other expert, work with what he has been given. The prospects of getting M to agree to make another recording in the expectation that he would obligingly switch accent during its progress were understandably remote, in any case. I therefore reported to the RUC that I was unable to give evidence that X and M were, or could be the same person, because such evidence would not have stood up for more than five minutes under cross-examination. There were certainly similarities, but the differences were such that only the assumption of accent-switching could account for them, and that assumption could not be justified on any principled grounds. As mentioned in the discussion of the case of J above, the RUC were obliged to pass on my opinion to the defence solicitor.

Naturally enough, he was delighted with the information, and, in due course, invited me to go to Belfast in order to discuss the case, and to make another recording of M. This was made necessary by the content of the earlier recorded interview, which included mention of M's previous prison record. In our system such information must be kept from the jury, whereas in other legal systems it could be looked on in quite a different light, namely as valuable information concerning the general character of the accused. It is a debatable point, of course: on the one hand our courts try to give maximal fairness to the accused by ensuring that each case is tried independently of any other, and on the other hand they suppress information regarding the accused's likelihood of having remained true to type, and committed the crime for which he is currently standing trial. I would prefer not to take a strong position on that controversy.

By this time M had been remanded in custody, and so it was necessary for me to visit him in prison in order to get a new sample of his speech which would be acceptable in court. He was very cooperative under those circumstances, since I was obviously acting in his best interests. He talked in an entirely relaxed way about his family background and childhood in Northern Ireland, and the sample was both substantial and clear. As I listened to him in the visiting room, where the recording was being made, it gradually began to register with me that his speech was very different from what it had been during the RUC interview. When I listened to the sample intensively later on that day I found that my immediate reactions were confirmed, and, furthermore, confirmed in every detail. All the features which had distinguished the speech of M from the speech of X were now absent - the glottal stops, the vowel qualities, the dental fricatives, etc., and I now had little doubt that X and M were, indeed, one and the same.

Under any system which is not so skewed in favour of the defence I would then have been asked to rejoin the prosecution and give evidence against M. That did not happen, of course. Since I had been passed over to the defence, and had agreed to act for them, I was irreversibly 'theirs'. Their options were few: they could discontinue with my evidence, accept that I was not going to be of very much help to them and release me, or they could ask me to appear in court, and give such evidence as defence counsel could devise to help his case. The latter option was taken, and I appeared in court for the defence. However, my evidence as led by counsel did not relate to the matter of identification, because, obviously, if I had been asked any questions about that aspect of the case, I would have had to give my opinion that the defendant M and the caller X were in all probability one and the same. Counsel had no doubts on this subject; when he was told my opinion by the solicitor his first words were, reportedly: 'Fucking hell! He thinks our man did it!'

His questions in my evidence-in-chief were on the very general matter of the ability of the layman to recognise live a voice he has only heard before on the telephone. My answer on that subject was that recognition of speakers by the layman is a mysterious operation, whether over the telephone or otherwise. The telephone system certainly introduced complicating factors by way of attenuating and distorting the message. Such recognition was not, therefore, reliable, and could be mistaken in any given instance. This was the totality of my evidence-in-chief. When prosecution counsel stood up I was fully expecting him to raise the matter of identification and the work I had done on it in this case. In fact, he did not do that, but confined himself to the topic of my evidence-in-chief. I was very surprised at that serious omission on his part, as it seemed to me at the time. I believe he was keeping strictly to the principle of cross-examination, which requires counsel to cross-examine only those matters raised in evidence-in-chief. Since identification of M with X had not been mentioned, there was no way in which he could have asked me questions about it.

The situation concerning evidence of identification in the case of M was this: I changed my earlier opinion from one favourable to the defence to one favourable to the prosecution on the basis of a further sample in which M showed accent-switching; this evidence could not be used by prosecution because I had already been transferred to the defence team; prosecution counsel could not raise the matter himself in court, since evidence is introduced by witnesses and not by counsel; my evidence-in-chief gave him no opportunity to do so in cross-examination. We thus found ourselves in a position in which evidence existed which could have been of significance to the court, but which was suppressed by the restrictive rules relating to evidence. As it happened in this case, prosecution had plenty of other evidence against M, and pursued the case successfully against him. It could well have been different, though. If, for instance, the evidence on speaker-identification had been more crucial in the case, the suppression of that evidence could have led to another outcome. I am sure that my experience here is not unique, but that there must have been many cases in our courts in which vital evidence for the prosecution failed to emerge for the reasons given above. It seems to me that the very worthy principle of equity is being misapplied in such cases, and that such undesirable, not to say ludicrous situations should motivate the relevant authorities to consider changing things. More will be said on this in Chapter 6.

As I mentioned above in passing, M was found guilty of attempting to gain money with menaces and with making threats to kill, and was sentenced to ten years in prison. I have had no further news of M, but I would not envy someone in his position. He was trying to exploit the very natural fear of terrorist organisations which exists in Northern Ireland for his own financial gain. As a freelance extortioner he was operating in a province in which extortion is the preserve of those terrorist organisations; they have been known to knee-cap, or worse, people who have, as they see it, usurped their authority. He was, if that was not already enough, making threats against a Roman Catholic family in the name, falsely, of the UVF, a Protestant terrorist organisation; this, again, would not be likely to endear him to that organisation in any event, but least of all as he was a Roman Catholic. Finally, as a Catholic himself he must have known full well the effect that such threats would have on the family he had selected as his victim.

It is very interesting to look at the motives for M's accent-switching. He adopted his Irish Irish version of his speech when in the interview with members of the RUC. He would assume, rightly or wrongly, that they were Protestants. They certainly all spoke with Scots Irish accents, and M obviously wanted to distance himself from them, probably both as individuals and as representatives of the RUC and, ultimately, the Crown. In his choice of accent he was identifying himself overtly with the Roman Catholic community, as well as with the Republicans and their aspirations. This is a very typical kind of reason for accent-switching.

Examining his reason for switching to a Scots Irish accent during his recorded interview with me, we find another common explanation. Asked by his solicitor why he had switched, he replied that he had done so in order to make himself more intelligible to me, an outsider. Ironically, by showing me that quite unnecessary consideration he had destroyed the major part of the defence case!

If M had not demonstrated that accent-switching was part of his normal behaviour in his own community, or if our courts permitted the use of tape-recordings in which the defendant's previous prison record is mentioned, I would have had no reason to change my opinion. I would have given evidence to the effect that I believed there was considerable doubt that M and X were the same person, since that was what I believed on the basis of the first M sample. Once the matter of speaker-identification had come out in court, though, the matter of accent-switching would have emerged also; even if that had not happened during my own presentation of evidence, it would have been the principal topic of any phonetics expert called by the prosecution in his evidence-in-chief, and in cross-examination by prosecution counsel I would have accepted the very lively possibility that such a thing could happen, and that, if it had, my conclusions could have been different. Again, this seems to me to be a somewhat ponderous, devious, and possibly unreliable means of introducing vital information to the court.

In my most recent case involving a charge of uttering threats to kill, I was contacted by a solicitor in Essex who was representing a man, let us call him Mr B, charged with that offence. The evidence against the man was that a woman, Mrs A, had received two anonymous telephone calls. Both calls were apparently by the same man, let us label him X, and in each her husband was threatened: in the first with having his legs blown off, and in the second with being killed. The woman was sure that Mr B had made both telephone calls.

The accused strenuously denied this. Neither of the calls had been recorded, and so the case against him depended on the evidence of recognition to be given by Mrs A. She had, it seems, known Mr B for some time in a social context, and had had substantial conversations with him on a number of occasions. She claimed, on the basis of those conversations, to have recognised the speech of Mr B over the telephone. The samples were not very long, but, as mentioned in the Introduction, length of sample does not appear to have much effect on the efficiency of the recognition process, whatever that may be. From this point of view, the case against Mr B was reasonably well-founded. However, Mrs A had never actually spoken with him over the telephone, and that was an important point in Mr B's favour.

Everyone must have noticed that we all sound different over the telephone. The reason for this is that the telephone-system changes the characteristics of the speech signal that it transmits to us by cutting out those frequencies which experience has shown are not vital to our understanding, usually those below about 100 Hz and above 4000 Hz. The band of frequencies that we do receive is enough to allow us to understand, usually, up to 100 per cent of the message, and it also contains all those features which are necessary for the forensic operation of speaker-identification.

When we listen to a voice 'live', we have access to the whole voice, i.e. all the frequency characteristics of that voice. As stated on more than one occasion above, the means by which speaker-recognition is carried out are unknown, but they must, obviously, refer to some characteristic(s) of that whole voice. If those characteristics are to be found predominantly or solely in the frequencies which are filtered out by the telephone system, the attenuated voice will sound different. Not only that, however. If the listener has not heard that voice before over the telephone, has not, therefore, had a chance to evolve a telephone recognition strategy specifically for it, the chances of that listener's recognising the voice are drastically reduced. The listener's hypothesised strategy must, of course, have been confirmed as successful on at least one occasion.

In the present case, Mrs A had never spoken with Mr B over the telephone, and, in consequence, could not claim that she could recognise him on that basis. She was claiming, however, that she could recognise him by his Essex accent, voice quality and intonation contours. She did not, of course, know the technical terms, but she expressed her points clearly enough. In doing so, she was referring to those very characteristics that would be considered by a phonetician in making a speaker-identification. They are all within the telephone version of the voice, and here, in fact, both speaker-recognition and identification coincide. As there were no recordings, there were no samples to be compared externally. Mrs A was making her own comparisons, but it was not possible, for obvious reasons, to tell whether they involved direct comparison of her auditory memory of Mr B's speech with her memory of the anonymous caller, or the comparison of both with some internal model. In any event, Mrs A's task would be made much easier if the speech of Mr B contained any salient features which she could then claim to have noticed in the speech of X.

This brings us to my second, though not subordinate role in the case. My first job was to provide the technical backup to the solicitor and eventually to the barrister engaged by Mr B. The second task was to carry out a phonetic analysis of the speech of Mr B to ascertain whether there were any salient features in it. I spoke to Mr B over the telephone, conversed over a cup of tea and recorded a long sample of his speech. In all, I had samples amounting to several thousand words. In analysing those samples, I found nothing in the least unusual; the voice quality was slightly breathy, the intonation contours were not exaggerated in either the over or under active sense, the rhythmic patterns and nucleus location were normal, the accent was typical of a male speaker of his age from Essex, in that there was rather more of London than of rural Essex in it. If Mrs A was going to claim in court that she could remember Mr B because of his idiosyncratic manner of speaking, then she was going to have difficulty in convincing me!

I attended the local magistrates' court in due course, and sat behind defence counsel while Mrs A was giving her evidence. From the sometimes anguished reaction of prosecution counsel it was obvious that she was presenting him with hitherto unheard items. For example, in her statement she had said that both calls were anonymous, whereas in court she remembered that in the first of them, X had identified himself by a name which she could not catch. That would have been one of the points defence counsel would have raised in cross-examination. He did not, however, get that far. In the purely routine matter of discovering if Mrs A could remember the dates of the calls, and if she had made any contemporaneous note to help her, inconsistencies emerged. She said that she did, in fact, have such a note (which was further news to prosecution counsel). When that note was produced, it was discovered that her record of the dates was totally different from the dates she had given in reporting the calls to British Telecom.

When prosecution added the effect on their case of these discrepancies to the evidence they knew I would be giving – that speaker-recognition cannot be relied on when the task is transferred from the live to the telephone context – they decided to withdraw the charge. Mr B was discharged and awarded full costs.

The case against Mr B was never very strong at best. Even if Mrs A had not unwittingly sabotaged it, I do not believe that it would have convinced the court because it was founded on the insubstantial evidence of auditory memory and speaker-recognition under unfavourable circumstances. Whilst driving back to London I had time to think about the way such flimsy evidence had been used as the basis of a criminal charge against

Mr B of uttering threats to kill. I could not help contrasting that case with another situation that I had been thinking about earlier in which threats to kill had also been uttered. Since that had been done in public and in England, not only the voices, but the faces and names and addresses of those who made those threats were known to the police. Yet, at the time of writing, no charge had been brought against those who threatened to kill, and/or incited others to kill Salman Rushdie. I was prompted to wonder why our legal system is perfectly capable of bringing such a charge, and on weak evidence, against people like Mr B, but is, apparently, unable to act in the case of those who publicly threatened the author.

Certainly the longest-running case in which I have been involved was the one described by the media at the time as the 'Christmas Tree' case. The investigation itself must have started substantially before that date, but as far as I was concerned, it all began in May 1982. The last rumblings, again, as far as I was involved, were in March 1987.

The Metropolitan Police were taking a close look at the minor criminal empire of John Goodwin, in much the same way as they had, some years earlier, examined the Krays' affairs. The police believed that two of their CID officers, a Detective Inspector L and a Detective Constable B, were implicated in the criminal affairs of John Goodwin. The were not 100 per cent sure of that, because they had no actual evidence. In order to secure information as to what the relationship was between those officers and Mr Goodwin, they persuaded an informant to conceal a miniature tape-recorder at the base of the Goodwins' Christmas Tree; the usual term for such a secret operation is to 'plant', but I do not believe such an instruction could have been interpreted literally at the time, because the resulting tape-recording was of excellent quality when I eventually heard it.

In May 1982 I received the tapes which were relevant to the case against the police officers. The Christmas Tree tape itself contained samples of the speech of five people; the uncontested speech of Mr Goodwin, that of two people alleged to be D/I L and D/C B, and the speech of two other people with whom I was not concerned. On this tape the speech sample of the alleged D/I L, let us label him ?D/I L, was both copious and clear. I was able to get a very full picture of his speech characteristics, both in its phonetic features and in its grammatical structures and vocabulary. The last two features, of course, were not part of the

phonetic analysis: any layman would have noticed constructions like 'We was', etc., and the speaker's frequent use of the
word 'shrewd', and that he was the only person in the conversation to use the word. Such observations could only become relevant as supporting indications in the event of an identification
having been made on purely phonetic grounds. No one would
conclude that two samples must have been spoken by the same
person because the word 'shrewd' was heard in both, not even
if there were some unusual pronunciation feature associated
with the word.

I have never actually encountered such a thing with a
favourite word, but I have with a problem word, i.e. a word
which the speaker always seemed to experience difficulty in
pronouncing. The case in question involved a Merseyside CID
officer who was the subject of an official complaints investigation by an outside police force, in this instance Greater
Manchester. Both the admitted and the contested samples were
good, and I had come to a pretty firm positive identification in
any case. What really made me convinced was the officer's
difficulty with the word 'solicitor'. Every time this word occurred in the admitted sample, four times in fact, he mispronounced it in a variety of ways – the most exotic of which could
be roughly rendered orthographically as 'sliztee'. I have no
explanation for this idiosyncracy; he was certainly not drunk,
for example, which is what I would have thought of as the most
likely cause. Whatever the reason, the same odd pronunciations
of this word cropped up three times in the contested sample. I
therefore felt as sure as I could be that the officer and the
alleged officer were the same person. I should, perhaps, repeat
the point made above to the effect that I would never give
primacy to such a word, however odd the pronunciation, over
phonetic comparison. I reported my opinion on identification
and in due course gave evidence in Liverpool Crown Court for
the prosecution. The officer was found guilty of soliciting bribes
and sentenced to three years in prison.

D/I L was interviewed by a senior police officer on some
general matter entirely unrelated to the affairs of Mr Goodwin.
Unknown to D/I L, that interview was being recorded on a
concealed tape-recorder, since his superiors had earlier come to
the conclusion that he would not be very likely to provide them
with a speech sample on a voluntary basis. When I compared
the phonetic characteristics of that sample with the one of ?D/I

L in the Christmas Tree tape, I found great similarity in all points of comparison. I also noted the use of the word 'shrewd' on a number of occasions, which gave further support to the positive identification. There were some differences between the samples in the matter of /h/-dropping, as well as in the extent to which the speakers' grammatical structures approximated to Standard English. There was far less /h/-dropping, and far fewer non-Standard constructions in the D/I L sample than in that of ?D/I L. A very remarkable feature in both samples was the occasional confusion of /v/ with /w/ in words like 'very' and 'wasn't', when the wrong one was used in each case. This was only sporadic in its occurrence, but throws a fascinating light on a feature of London speech which people tend to believe has either died out, after the passing of the generation of Dickens's 'Sam Weller', or never really existed in the first place.

Weighing the discrepancies against the overwhelming similarities mentioned above, I felt that it was much more likely that the former were due to a probably unconscious adjustment of his speech habits by the same speaker to the more formal context of an interview by a senior officer, than they were indications that the two samples had been spoken by different people. Taking everything into consideration, I was as sure as I could be that D/I L and ?D/I L were in fact the same person.

When I listened to the sample of the alleged D/C B, i.e. ?D/C B, on the Christmas Tree tape, I found a number of problems in describing it phonetically. For one thing, this speaker did not say as much in the conversations as did ?D/I L, and of those contributions he did make, he whispered a substantial proportion. Some utterances which had the general pitch and rhythmic characteristics of his speech could not be understood, and, of course, no phonetic analysis can be made of unintelligible utterances. I did finally succeed in building up an adequate picture of his speech, at the cost of much time and effort. Two interesting features of his accent that I noted were, first: the frequent realisation of /k/ and /g/ as very retracted, almost uvular when they occurred before non-front vowels, and second: the occasional incidence of 'consonant capture'. This term refers to the process whereby a consonant which occurs at the end of a word is 'captured' by a following word if that word begins with a vowel, as in 'and eliminated' → 'an deliminated', or 'brought out' → 'brough tout'. The difference between the two can clearly be perceived on the basis of durational and other phonetic features, the details of which need not concern the general reader. In London speech there is generally a markedly different allophone of the same vowel phoneme in words like 'pour' and 'port', depending on whether that vowel occurs word-finally or not. It is important to note that the word-final allophone does not occur in 'brough' as a result of such consonant capture. This phenomenon is heard fairly often from speakers with a very marked London accent, but by no means all such speakers do it, so it does add weight to a positive identification when it occurs.

The last process does not appear to be typical of English in general, though I believe it can occur in a certain type of Glaswegian accent. It is, however, a regular, indeed an obligatory feature of many other languages, including French. In the case of the present speaker, and in all the other speakers I have observed carrying out this process, there has never been any demonstrable French connection, unless, in the case of families which have lived very many generations in London, particularly East London, there could be a Huguenot substratum. I must confess to the reader at this point that reference to an untestable 'substratum' is often made by linguists by way of explanation for phenomena which otherwise elude explanation, and that, in consequence, they should not place too much reliance on its appropriateness here.

As in the case of D/I L, a senior officer interviewed D/C B, and, once again, the conversation was recorded. In comparing this sample with that of ?D/C B I found correspondences on every point of comparison, including and especially of those unusual features mentioned above. I was able to conclude that both samples had, in my opinion, been spoken by the same person, i.e. D/C B.

I submitted my report on both officers to the same effect, and on the basis of this and other evidence they were charged with conspiracy and suspended from duty. Both men maintained throughout the case that they were not guilty. I reported at the beginning of July 1982, but the first court hearing was not until the middle of July 1983. This was in a magistrates' court, and took the form of an 'old style' committal. This kind of committal is held at the request of defence, who can then ask for any or all of the prosecution's evidence to be presented. When they have heard it, they can make a submission that there is no case to answer, and that further proceedings should be abandoned.

On this occasion, as far as I was aware, they elected to call all the prosecution witnesses, including me. My evidence was meticulously written down and my notes examined by the defence. They seemed to be particularly interested in two non-phonetic notes I had made at the end of my phonetic summary. I had written down 'an invicative position' and 'if my plans come to fruitition'. They acted with extreme, almost comic suspicion towards these notes, carefully checking the spelling with me of the non-existent words, but failed to ask me why I had written them down. I could have told them that there was no mystery, I had simply noted the utterances as being of interest to me because they were typical of the speech of an ambitious and pretentious, but uneducated person like Mr Goodwin. They had absolutely nothing to do with the case against the police officers, or, indeed, anyone else.

I fully expected these phrases to re-appear at the next court hearing, but they did not. That did not take place until April 1984, in the Central Criminal Court (Old Bailey). At the end of that trial, in which I gave the same evidence as at the committal, the jury found D/I L guilty, but D/C B innocent. It had been argued on behalf of the latter that he had taken part in the conversations, but had said nothing of an incriminating nature. Looking at his utterances in the transcript, that was certainly a reasonable argument. He was not, after all, on trial for associating with known criminals, or even for being in the same room when criminal acts were being planned, but for conspiracy, and that charge depended on what he could be heard to say on the Christmas Tree tape. The fact that he whispered many of his utterances on that tape so that they could not be heard, could not, of course, be held against him - there could have been a perfectly innocent reason for his speaking in that way.

D/I L was sentenced to two years imprisonment. He left prison to attend his disciplinary hearing in Tintagel House at the end of September 1985, at which, again, I gave evidence. The hearing found against him, with all the implications that entailed.

The last time I saw D/I L was also in Tintagel House, at a Secretary of State's Tribunal in March 1987. This latter institution is the highest appeal court available to a police officer; as in all the other hearings, this one too found against him, and upheld the conclusions of the disciplinary hearing. Since the weight of evidence had always been overwhelmingly against him, I cannot see how he could have entertained any hopes of success in his appeal, but he tried nevertheless. It is possible that he felt it necessary to make a gesture, although the nature of the gesture, if indeed that is what it was, remains obscure.

In a different case involving a police officer on a charge of corruption, the accused steadfastly pleaded 'not guilty' throughout his lengthy old-style committal proceedings, and continued to do so at his trial in the Central Criminal Court. At least, that is, until day two of that trial, when, without prior warning, he changed his plea to one of 'guilty'. I have tried to think what his motive for that sudden change of heart might have been. One explanation is that he genuinely 'saw the light' whilst sitting in court that morning, and realised that the only honest and proper course for him was to plead 'guilty'. It would be unwise to discount the possibility of such a revelation happening in even the apparently most unpromising individual, and I sincerely hope that that is the true reason for his volte face. However, other explanations present themselves. The timing of his change of plea may not have been providential. He had gone through the most elaborate procedures available to him in the conduct of his case up to and including his Old Bailey trial. There the timing of his change of plea incurred the maximum inconvenience and expense for the authorities, and, potentially, the maximum advantage for himself.

In the first place, as a police officer in London he must have had a very good idea of the complications involved in assembling and co-ordinating witnesses. He must also have had some notion of the cost of running an old-style committal followed by a trial at the Central Criminal Court; according to a recent un-official estimate, the latter now costs £45 a *second*!

In the second place he could still perhaps have hoped to secure the lighter sentence which a plea of 'guilty' often encourages, although in his case that may have been misplaced optimism, since the judge would undoubtedly have been fully aware of the implications of his action, and could have felt that the defendant was trying to exploit the convention. The possibility of a less charitable explanation cannot, unfor-tunately, be denied: the defendant's pattern of pleading was motivated by sheer malice.

The last act in the Christmas Tree saga, again one in which I gave evidence of identification for the prosecution, was a case of kidnapping, or 'unlawful imprisonment' in the legal phrasing. Whilst John Goodwin was in prison as a result of the present case, it occurred to some of his erstwhile associates that he must have salted away large amounts of 'hot' money. Mr Goodwin had been involved in a considerable number of major robberies, and they reasoned that, as a prudent and successful operator, he must have kept concealed from the police investigation much of his share of the booty. They further reasoned that he must have told his wife the details of any secret accounts, and the like, so that she could keep an eye on things until he came out of prison. They needed to find a way of extracting the information from Mrs Goodwin, and took what was to them the obvious step: they kidnapped her. She was placed under constant threat of physical violence, and I believe she was actually assaulted. She was interrogated at great length by the chief of her captors about the money her husband had received from the robberies, and also about the personnel who had worked with him on some of the jobs. She must have managed to convince him that she really did not know anything abut secret money, even assuming it existed in the first place, and also that her marriage to John Goodwin was effectively over, because she was released.

Eventually, in October 1985, one man who had pleaded 'not guilty' to a number of charges, including that of 'unlawful imprisonment', was brought to trial at the Old Bailey. An informer, who had co-operated with the police, had smuggled a tape-recorder into the house where Mrs Goodwin was being held, and much of her interrogation had been recorded. I compared the speech of the interrogator with that of a suspect in interviews with police officers, and could find no phonetic differences between them. I gave evidence to that effect. The accused was found 'guilty' on all the charges, and was sentenced to 14 years in prison. This case leads us into the next, which will be the last that I am going to describe, because it, too, was one in which the defendant was accused of 'unlawful imprisonment'.

The case of R went to trial at the end of November 1989 in Southwark Crown Court, London, and was, therefore, my last major trial before the deadline of *Forensic Phonetics*. For that reason alone it would have been a logical candidate for inclusion in this selection, bearing in mind that the present Chapter 5 began with my first case. As it transpired, the nature of this case, together with the way in which certain aspects of it were conducted, brought the role of the expert in the adversarial legal system into particularly sharp focus, and I would have found it essential to include it in any event.

A number of men probably most fairly described as 'adventurers' came together in a plan to kidnap a wealthy Arab doctor resident in London, and to hold him hostage against payment of a substantial ransom by his family. The Anti-Terrorist Branch of New Scotland Yard believe there could have been as many as ten men involved in the conspiracy. The identities of, probably, four men remained unclear throughout the investigation, but the particulars of six alleged conspirators were known to the police, including that of the man they believed was the ringleader, R. My involvement in the case was solely with the last, who pleaded 'not guilty' to the charge of 'conspiring with others unlawfully to imprison and detain against his will' the victim. Of the five other known suspects, one, an Arab, was reportedly detained in Syria, whilst the remaining four pleaded 'guilty' in English courts, and were given relatively light sentences.

I am describing the case of R principally because of its importance in airing a number of controversies in the world of forensic phonetics, and do not, therefore, propose to take the reader through all the details of the progress of the investigation, although that would make a good story on another occasion. One item I would like to include here, though, is that at the very time the alleged R was instructing the victim's family on how to pay the ransom, the victim himself had succeeded in escaping from his captors, and was on his way home! No ransom, of course, was ever paid.

The recorded speech sample of R took the form of a video-cassette in which he was introducing a group of young men to the mysteries of an outdoor 'war-game' course which he ran, quite legitimately and, apparently, successfully. This sample consisted of many hundreds of words, and, despite its location, was for the most part very clear. The ?R samples consisted of several telephone calls to the victim's family, and also a large number of calls to a car-hire firm, the services of which ?R tried to commission to pick up the suitcases containing, as he hoped and supposed, the ransom. When there are multiple unknown samples, as in this case, the phonetician's first job is to ascertain whether they can be treated, in his opinion, as one composite sample, or whether there seems to be more than one speaker. On this occasion I had little difficulty in deciding that there was only one speaker. This sample, too, was very long, and mostly clear.

Comparison of the samples revealed very close similarities in the features of voice quality, pitch and intonation. In terms of both the phonemic systems and the realisations of the phonemes I could find no differences; both R and ?R showed occasional traces of a semi-rhotic accent, for example, and there was comparable variation in the realisations of /r/ by both speakers, in that they each used approximant and tap in about equal proportion. I found the same kind of similarity in every aspect of comparison. The sporadic attempts by ?R at an American accent were ludicrously inconsistent and transparent, and there were no other discrepancies that I could discover. I therefore reported that I was as sure as I could be that R and ?R were the same person.

On the basis of this and other evidence, R was arrested and charged as described in an earlier paragraph. Since the major prop of the prosecution case against R was my evidence of identification, it was certain that defence would find a phonetics expert of their own. Their first hope would be that he or she would be able to find flaws in my comparisons, and thereby to counter them in court. Defence elected for an old-style committal, and I discovered that they had indeed consulted such an expert, a phonetician from Cambridge University, who was present in court during that committal. I gave my evidence-in-chief in the customary manner, and waited expectantly for junior defence counsel to reveal in his cross-examination the line they would be taking in the case. It became clear to me as he proceeded that they were not going to take issue with my conclusions, since no questions were put to me on that aspect of my evidence. Obviously, their expert had carried out his own phonetic comparisons of the samples, and had come to the same conclusion as I had. This became even more certain when defence did not call their expert to give evidence. In this kind of situation, when the expert first consulted by the defence has come up with the 'wrong' opinion, it is often the case that they will 'shop around' in the hopes of finding another expert who will oblige by coming to the 'right' conclusion. On this occasion they did not do that because they had reason to believe that they would still be able to use their expert's professional advice as the basis of an attack, not on my conclusions, but on my methods.

In Chapter 1 – Introduction I said that it is my belief that phonetic comparisons for forensic purposes can be carried out on a purely auditory basis, and I tried to explain my reasons for saying that. I also mentioned that this is a matter of some controversy, and that not all phoneticians agree with my position. One form of dissent is the opinion held by the Cambridge expert that auditory analysis is neither accurate nor efficient enough to stand on its own; his view is that such examination must be backed up, i.e. its findings confirmed, by acoustic analysis. He feels particularly strongly that evidence of identification carried out solely on the auditory basis should not be permitted in courts in this country. Whilst acting for the defence in an earlier case, he had made certain discoveries which convinced him, at least, on this point. (The case in question is mentioned in Chapter 3 – Acoustic Phonetics.) When he was consulted by the defence in the present case he must have welcomed it as an opportunity to attack the auditory method in court.

Although there were one or two questions about the differences between the two methods then, that attack did not come during the committal. Defence clearly needed more time to prepare their ground, and the months which elapsed between the committal and the Crown court hearing gave them more than enough in which to do so.

At the Crown Court, defence was led, not by junior counsel, but by leading counsel, and he was able to present a thoroughly well-researched case, thanks largely to my Cambridge colleague, against the auditory method. His first move was to submit to the court that my evidence was not of an 'expert' character, and that it should be excluded. This required, as usual, a trial-within-a-trial. During a cross-examination lasting all of one day, defence counsel put every conceivable argument to me against the auditory method, whilst I held to the arguments I have already presented in the Introduction. At the end of these proceedings the judge decided that I was, in his view, an expert, and that my evidence should be heard before the jury.

In the trial proper, defence counsel put more or less the same arguments to me in cross-examination as in the trial-within-a-trial, with some innovations. The chief of these was that he not only sought to destroy the validity of the auditory method, but to attack my personal integrity and honesty. He asked if I took the oath one swears in court seriously, and accused me of habitually breaking that oath by deliberately misleading juries, in that I did not tell them that my evidence is fallible. I explained to the jury that I always make this particular point clear, i.e. that no method of speaker-identification is 100 per cent sure, that we cannot look on any identification based on phonetic analysis and comparison as being certain in the way it could be when finger-print comparisons are involved, as so on.

Re-examination did not take very long. Prosecution counsel asked if I had already said many times in cross-examination that one of the most important controls on the efficiency and the validity of the auditory method was that it could be checked by other phoneticians, including those who favoured the auditory/ acoustic approach. I agreed that this was so. She then asked if I had seen in court another phonetics expert during my evidence-in-chief and cross-examination. I said that I had (though he was not present in court that morning). Next she asked where he had been sitting – 'Behind defence counsel'.

'What is his approach in forensic phonetics?'

'He is a specialist in the auditory/acoustic approach.'

'What is his name?', to which I gave the appropriate answer. That concluded the case for the prosecution.

I had to leave the court at that point, and so was not present during the closing speeches by counsel or the judge's summing-up. What happened next was reported to me later. There were no witnesses for the defence; my Cambridge colleague had disappeared by then, and the defendant was not called to speak on his own behalf. The jury duly retired after the judge's summing-up to consider their verdict. All those most closely involved in the case remained in the courthouse to await the jury's verdict, many having a much-needed cup of coffee. The courtroom was taken over by another trial, probably for the purpose of sentencing, since that would not normally take very long, and the courtroom would be free for as long as it took the jury to make up their minds. After *five minutes* a knock was heard from the jury room, and the usher responsible for the care of the jury assumed they needed to clarify some point of law, or that they had some other problem. In fact, the foreman of the jury told the usher that they had reached their verdict! (I have been told that this may be a record in brevity.) He told the jury that they could not return to the courtroom until its present occupants had finished their business, which they did about fifteen minutes later. The surprised participants in R's case returned, their coffees unfinished, to hear the jury's verdict 'guilty, and unanimously so'. The judge had the final word in sentencing R to ten years in prison. I understand that defence have asked for leave to appeal, but I do not know on what grounds.

The conduct of this case raises some important issues in respect of the expert's role, particularly when he is acting for the defence. In the absence of any real case in the form of witnesses or alibi, or any evidence against the substance of my identification, the only course open to defence counsel was to attempt to invalidate my method. In the first place this was attempted in the trial-within-a-trial, but without success. In the trial proper, counsel once more attacked my method, knowing full well that his own expert had confirmed the effectiveness of it in this instance. He also attacked my integrity as an academic and my honesty in presenting my evidence, not only on that occasion, but on all such occasions in the past. He was able to make the preposterous allegation of my dishonesty when he had his own expert sitting within yards of him who knew full well that that was not so.

Defence counsel's case was obviously parlous, and his only hope of success was to try to destroy my evidence, which he is, of course, perfectly entitled to do. Ironically, the more he denigrated my method and exaggerated the effectiveness of the method I had not used, the auditory/acoustic method, the more he was setting himself up for prosecution counsel's coup de grace. I was able to identify an expert in his much-vaunted method who had been present in court the whole time, but had not been called to explain to the jury where I was mistaken in my evidence. Every argument against me on this subject was a coffin-nail in his own case, because he must have raised the jury's expectations that such refuting evidence would be produced, which he then failed to deliver. I find it hard to account for counsel's personal attack on me. It could be that he knew his only hope lay in breaking me as a witness, and that he allowed his desperation and frustration to get the better of him. I had understood it to be a principle of cross-examination of expert witnesses that their methods and conclusions could be attacked, but that gratuitous slurs on their personal and professional honesty were beyond the pale. This was not, in fact, the first such occurrence in my career, and it is possible, therefore, that it is I who am mistaken. Another explanation could be that defence counsel genuinely believes that behaviour of that sort is laudable; if my experience of him is typical, and if we remember that he is a QC, it can only be concluded that he has won respect and recognition in his profession on the basis of that kind of conduct. I will leave the reader to draw his or her own inferences on that. As far as counsel's attempting to confuse the jury was concerned, their comment on it was far more telling than anything I could say. They had followed his argument step by step as it proceeded, and they arrived at the unanimous conclusion that defence counsel was transparently wrong. Furthermore, they arrived at that conclusion in record time!

I find certain aspects of the role of the expert consulted by defence in this case to be regrettable. When he was first approached by defence and asked to help then in the case, he must have accepted in the knowledge that I had used the auditory method. Since, as I have said above, he believes strongly that that approach is not valid, he must have entertained hopes that he would be able to demonstrate its shortcomings in open court. I have no doubt that he carried out every possible test in comparing the samples, and at the end of those exhaustive operations he must have arrived at the unexpected, possibly disappointing conclusion that my opinion was correct within his own terms of reference. He then co-operated with defence in preparing a bitter assault on the auditory method. He was thus put in the curious, (not to say 'invicative') position (as John Goodwin would have had it), of witnessing an attack in court on the efficiency of a method which he himself had confirmed as efficient, even if he only believed that to be a fluke. He was invited by prosecution to go into the witness-box and to give his opinions in an objective manner, i.e. to explain his objections to the method I had used, and to say, if he wished, that I had got it right on this occasion more by luck than judgment. He declined this invitation, however. I can only conclude that his enthusiasm to see the auditory method attacked by counsel outweighed his interest in giving the court the benefit of his own opinions in person. I find this particularly regrettable. Our system does not seem to require the expert to be impartial, but surely it is not unreasonable to hope that he will make every effort to be so, and not set winning above the truth in a given case, however important he may believe his ulterior motives to be.

Had defence counsel succeeded in convincing the jury that the method I had used was fallacious, and had they found R 'not guilty', the latter would have gone free. Counsel would no doubt have congratulated himself on securing, against all the odds, the acquittal of a man concerning whom all the evidence was in agreement, including the expert opinion substantiated by his own expert. This would have been properly in accordance with our law, but justice in the general sense would not, surely, have been served. Nor would it have been served in a narrower sense; if the victim and his family had any moral right to see punished within our legal system the man who had caused them so much distress, that right would have been denied them.

Chapter 6

The Future

The many controversies in the business of speaker-identification by means of phonetic analysis and comparison which have been discussed in the preceeding pages would all, probably, entirely disappear if there really were such a thing as a 'voice-print'. Although it does not exist at the moment, I would certainly not wish to rule out the possibility that such a thing might be developed in the course of time. I would like, in fact, to put it on record that I positively believe there will one day be a 'voice-print', i.e. a print-out from some sort of, not necessarily electronic, device which will be able uniquely to identify an individual speaker. I am basing this belief on the premises that each human vocal tract is unique, both in its configurations and in its sound outputs, and that the technical resources now available for acquiring, storing and matching data on those matters are primitive in the extreme. When I have mentioned this prediction to colleagues, I have encountered various responses; some do not think it will ever be technically feasible, whilst others express varying measures of agreement. One, the head of the Speaker-Identification Unit of the Federal Criminal Bureau in West Germany, was the most sanguine, saying that he certainly believed there would eventually be such a thing, but that it could not be expected in less than twenty years. He believed that the necessary advance of technology would take at least that long. I am not a scientist, or computer specialist, and cannot, therefore, claim to be able to give an informed opinion from within the field. However, it seems to me, an interested observer, that computer technology is advancing, not step-by-step in a laboriously unilinear fashion, not even geometrically, but multi-dimensionally. I do not, consequently, think it possible to put a minimal time limit on anything which necessarily involves so many variables and unpredictables; I would not be in the least surprised to see a real 'voice-print' in the not too distant future.

If and when such a resource exists, it follows that it will supercede other methods of speaker-identification, including, naturally, my own. I remember the reaction of amazement and disbelief when, in cross-examination, I volunteered the same opinion to defence counsel in the case of R (Chapter 5). He apparently found it hard to believe that any expert could with equanimity predict the surplanting of his own expertise by the progress of science. I sincerely hope that this difficulty is simply the product of the low esteem in which that individual seems to hold experts, and that it is not shared by too many others in his profession.

As I envisage it, future developments of computer technology will produce machines which will be vastly faster than those now available. I believe there is some possibility that future computers could leave their base in electronics, and move to a light-based system. This would have the advantage of operating at something approaching the speed of light. Tasks which still take computers a long while to 'chug' their way through would be completed in a fraction of that time. There is also the possibility of a vastly-expanded storage capacity, perhaps even moving in the direction of the infinite. The data-base would be accessed readily enough by the high-speed computer, and this would not necessarily be a binary system. If it were n-ary it would permit cross-referencing of the data, which, again, would offer enormous resources.

I would imagine the identification process to begin with the inputting of a speech sample. The analysis would probably still need to be given a general orientation with categories like 'human', 'male', 'child' and so on, exhausting the fund of existing knowledge or beliefs about the speaker, in order to reduce the number of hypotheses the machine is asked to check. The human element here in controlling and directing the machine will, I am sure, always be essential. The machine's first task would be to provide a model, or a series of models in diminishing order of probability, of the vocal tract(s) which could have produced the sounds. The second task would be to match that model against other models stored in the system. Each of these tasks would still require an astronomical number of operations to be performed. Whilst it is true that present devices cannot handle such astronomical quantities, for a machine which itself operates at astronomical speeds on astronomical data-bases, the same problems would obviously not present themselves.

The results of the comparison would be presented in such terms as 'a complete match', i.e. a 100 per cent certain identification, or it could be a 'resemblance' to a specific order of probability. 'Different speakers' would, of course, be the third category. If a print-out of the computer models were required, I would suppose that to be in some kind of holographic form. I would suggest the term 'vocal-tract print', since that seems to describe more accurately what I envisage the actual product of the machine to be.

These ideas may seem, to some readers at least, to be much more related to science-fiction than to any kind of foreseeable reality. My answer to that objection is to point out that, not many decades ago, most of the electronic resources now commonly available were themselves firmly in the realm of fiction, to say nothing of 'men on the moon'. As I said earlier, I believe that progress in computer technology, as well as in other forms of technology, will accelerate for a long time yet, and I have no doubt that the 'voice-print', or rather, the 'vocal-tract print', will have been made possible long before such progress levels off, if indeed it ever does.

Until such things are possible, though, we have to make the best of what we have by way of speaker-identification, etc., and that means using the procedures outlined in the preceding pages. I have tried to make it clear to the reader that I am sure that the English adversarial system, in my experience of it, fails to make the best of what we have. That remains true, too, if one looks at it from the point of view of cost-effectiveness. The case of R is a good example of what I mean. From the time the defence expert produced his report that he agreed with my findings, the story is consistently one of waste; waste in the form of fees to the professionals, time spent waiting in court by police and others as required by the system when they could have been doing something more productive elsewhere, the vast outlay of expenditure needed to stage both the old-style committal and the Crown court trial, and so on. There is, too, the further cost of an appeal, if that should be permitted. All of this in the cause of staging a confrontation between two sides, prosecution and defence, on the entirely spurious argument that defence counsel might find some loophole in the prosecution case. His only hope of such a breakthrough depended on his suppressing inconvenient evidence.

This is, of course, perfectly 'honest' within our system, but simply could not happen in an 'inquisitorial' system of the kind generally found in Europe, and, nearer home, in Scotland. This aspect of our legal system is far from being the object of admiration in other countries that some people complacently expect or suppose it to be. When I have described the sort of things mentioned in the earlier pages to colleagues who work within different systems, their reactions range from incredulity and shock, through bafflement to contempt (depending on their general opinions of the English). The one reaction I have yet to encounter is that of any kind of approval, or even comprehension. I do not attempt to defend our system to those colleagues, because I believe that it is fundamentally misconceived; if it were possible, I would like to suggest a thorough re-think of the philosophy underlying that system, with the strong requirement that it be re-done according to what I and many other academics see as rational principles. Looking at it practically, though, I know that such a revolution cannot be brought about. I would, consequently, be only too happy to settle for some movement towards the elimination of, at least, the most embarrassing, costly and illogical of its features.

One step in the right direction would be the removal of the expert and his evidence from the adversarial domain. In most countries in Europe the expert is consulted by the court, and is expected to present his opinion in an impartial manner. He is required to tell the court everything he has found, with, naturally, no editing or suppression of information. What the expert has concluded becomes, thus, the common property of all those involved in the case, and there can be no secrets. He can, of course, be questioned quite rigorously by any relevant party, but could not be subjected to the kind of discourtesy probably all experts have met with in English courts. Such personal attacks are totally out of place in a rational environment, where the objective is to discover all the relevant facts. Where there is a dispute about the facts, a second, or even a third opinion may be obtained, and a number of arguments set before the court. I believe it is possible for experts to agree to a compromise position with respect to their joint statement presented to the court.

All of this seems very sensible to me, and I know that many of my colleagues in the academic world feel similarly. I speak for them also when I say that I would very much like to see some comparable arrangement in England. It is possible that more phoneticians would come forward to assist a 'court of inquiry', which they perceive as rational, as opposed to the irrationality of our present system. Also, they might not always feel very happy about facing the to them unnecessary and avoidable stresses and pressures of the adversarial system. Naturally, not everyone would welcome such a change; I would suppose that many defence specialists would, probably, react with horror at this proposed removal of one of their mainstays in court – the right to suppress evidence.

As an example, we might consider how such a revised system would have operated in the case of R. A 'court of inquiry' would have heard submissions from both experts at a lower level, possibly an appropriately modified magistrates' court. Both their disagreement as to method and their agreement as to identification of R would have been recorded, as would the other evidence of identification presented in the case. Where there is unanimity of evidence at that level (remember, there were no witnesses for the defence), one cannot possibly justify the removal of the case to a higher court. The reader will recall that some considerable time had been spent at the Crown court by defence before the trial proper, trying to convince the judge that my evidence was not 'expert'. This is seen by my colleagues, Continental and domestic, and by myself as a totally vacuous exercise, since the Cambridge expert had come to the same conclusion as I had on the identification of R with ?R. A rational system would eliminate such operations, thereby saving an enormous sum of money, and relieving the court of the task of laboriously working its way through defence counsel's arguments to arrive at what was, in my opinion, a foregone conclusion.

As I understand the situation at present, some cases are automatically sent for trial at the higher level because of the seriousness of the charge(s) in legal convention, and the case of R is a typical example. There are many occasions, however, when that does not seem to be the case, and the decision to be tried at the higher level depends on the wish of the accused. I believe the exercising of this option to be the principle cause of the delay between committal and trial, at least a year at the present time, and the near-terminal congestion of cases waiting to be heard in the Crown courts.

The wastefulness of this aspect of the system can be exemplified by the following case. I was recently required to attend a Crown court in a case in which a young man was accused of having made a number of obscene telephone calls to a businessman. Threats to kill had also been uttered. I had made a statement to the effect that I believed the accused to have been responsible for those calls. Other experts for the prosecution were also called to the court, and the whole mechanism of a Crown court trial was set under way. The defendant then announced that he would plead 'guilty', since the expert consulted by defence agreed with my opinion. This case had been taken through a normal committal at the magistrates' court, in which no evidence had been heard, and, at the accused's request, sent for trial by jury in the Crown court, with the outcome I have just described. Whatever the outcome, it seems to me quite wrong in principle that such a case should not have been dealt with at the magistrates' level; once again, there would have been a great economy of resources, and no lack of justice, since that level is perfectly well-equipped to deal with such cases. I do not think the accused should exercise the right to trial by jury; it seems to me more logical to have two clear categories of case, which would be tried without equivocation on either the higher or the lower level.

What I am suggesting here would entail the upgrading of the present magistrates' courts. This could be done, I think, by the establishment of a post of, say, 'chairman of the magistrates', who would be a senior lawyer or barrister. The other members of the court would continue to be non-legal people. Possibly an increase in the number of lay magistrates sitting would be considered desirable, perhaps to four. This re-constituted court would hear:

- minor cases (as it now does);
- any case in which there is unanimity of evidence;
- any case in which there is a plea of 'guilty'.

It would, naturally, need to be empowered to sentence to the highest level permitted by the law. A further vital function of such a court would be to hear expert evidence as a 'court of inquiry'. Only if the case were both serious and contentious would it be transferred to the Crown court; the function of the lower court in that event would be to transmit an agreed expert statement to the higher court. If the opinions of the experts cancelled one another out, this information would be handed on to the Crown court, but in neither event would the experts give their evidence in the latter. If any questions were to arise in the

Crown court about the statement of expert opinion, the judge, together with counsel, would call such experts as they considered necessary to give clarification to them, in the absence of the jury. I have suggested excluding the personal presentation of expert evidence from the Crown court because I believe it should properly be dealt with in the 'court of inquiry', which would, by definition, exclude what I consider to be the most serious defect of the adversarial system: its emphasis on winning the case as opposed to discovering the truth. Those barristers with a penchant for winning defence cases would, I am sure, continue to find ample outlets for their talents at the Crown court level, where the adversarial system would probably prove to be too deeply entrenched to be eradicated.

Another effect of the revisions proposed above would be to transfer the burden of assessing highly complex expert evidence from the jury to the 'court of inquiry'. It would be the latter's task, if the case were transferred, to hand on to the Crown court jury the results of that assessment, which would include summaries of the evidence and some statement of probabilities for the jury's guidance. All of this communication would, most essentially, be couched in plain English, so that the jurymen would not have to guess at what was meant by it. An important advantage of this method would be that it would leave the principle of 'trial by jury', as opposed to 'trial by experts', intact, and would, in fact, render juries more capable of dealing with such evidence by pre-digesting the most difficult parts of it. The jury would, therefore, still draw their own conclusions on that category of evidence, but I would contend that they would do so in a more informed way in such a revised system.

There is the further possibility that a jury could be swayed by a charismatic presenter to accept what might be weak evidence on his part, and to reject sound evidence from a dull presenter. A good performance is not evidence, I believe. I know this is something the judge would try to make clear to the jury when necessary, but the removal of expert evidence from the Crown court would obviate that necessity. With all due respect to those who serve on juries, a professionalised 'court of inquiry' would, I think, be far less susceptible to such superficially attractive arguments.

I realise that I have offended against tradition and practice in many of the criticisms and suggestions I have made; I would plead 'fair comment' here, since I have not written against anything, the significance of which my own direct experience has not given me good cause to reflect on. I feel very strongly that the time is ripe for a more substantial move forward in our legal system. I am encouraged in this belief by the efforts recently made to update certain aspects of that system, and even more so by our imminent entry into a much closer relationship with our neighbours in Europe. I believe that we, as a nation, are mature enough to accept improvement and rationalisation in some of our most hallowed institutions (such as our legal system), modelled on practices elsewhere, just as we would hope to be able to provide a sensible input into processes of change in other countries. With regard, specifically, to forensic phonetics, practitioners in Britain are looking forward to working in closer co-operation with their colleagues in Europe. Although they are still on an unofficial basis, we have already established contacts, which we hope will develop into fruitful collaboration, with our colleagues in forensic phonetics in West Germany and the Netherlands. We would hope, in the future, to extend these contacts wherever feasible in Europe.

Notes

Chapter 1

1. 'Ear-training' as a method of developing the auditory skills of phonetics students was initiated by Daniel Jones during his head-ship of the Department of Phonetics at University College London. 'Words' are dictated to the student consisting of sounds of the student's own language, or including the sounds of any known language. There is the further possibility that sounds from no known language can be introduced. The student writes down his judgements about the sounds he has heard by means of the symbols of the International Phonetic Alphabet. This is a tried and tested method of instruction which is now used in any institution in which practical phonetics is taught in a serious way.
2. When a trial-within-a-trial is held, the witness may already have taken the general oath mentioned, and in that case there is no further requirement for an oath to be taken. If, however, no oath has been taken, I believe the correct oath under those circumstances to be: 'I swear by Almighty God that I will truthfully answer any questions the court may ask of me'.

Chapter 2

1. There are many institutions, both in Europe and elsewhere, which give instructions on how to pronounce the sounds of a language to native speakers of that language. Such institutions do not normally function as advisory bodies, giving advice when asked for it, but rather as authorities giving instructions which they expect to be obeyed. Probably the best known of these is the Académie Française in the case of French, but something very similar was done for German by Siebs at the turn of the century. In the Soviet Union the Academy of Sciences states unequivocally the rules governing the standard pronunciation of Russian, and sternly warns that any deviation from those norms will be perceived as 'linguistically uncultured'.

2. When he was establishing the validity of phonetics as an academic subject, Daniel Jones was particularly well-aware of the damage that prescriptivism could have done to his efforts, and he avoided it at all costs. The following story illustrates that point. I have not been able to discover any documentary evidence in support of it, and must, therefore, present it as part of the folk-lore of Gordon Square. It seems that George Bernard Shaw wanted Daniel Jones to set up a unit in UCL to prescribe a standard pronunciation for English, and offered to leave a substantial sum of money in his will to finance it. Jones was horrified at this suggestion, and rejected the offer, no doubt trying to explain the difference between 'descriptive' and 'prescriptive' to Shaw. The latter cannot have been impressed, because he left the money instead to run a competition for a 'new English alphabet'. The cash prize was duly won, and, as instructed posthumously by Shaw, a limited edition of 'Androcles and the Lion' was printed in the prize-winning alphabet. Since that time, nothing more has been heard of the alphabet, and it is probably true to say that Shaw did the equivalent of pouring his money down the drain. The 'GBS Memorial Lectureship', or whatever, which Jones could have set up at UCL under more rational circumstances, never came into existence.

Chapter 4

1. All matters relating to Speech Therapy - examinations, statistics, Parliamentary questions, etc. - are monitored by the College of Speech Therapists in London, and I shall in consequence comment only briefly here. The Quirk Report of 1972 recommended that there should be 6 Speech Therapists per 100,000 of the population. Central Government has no policy in this matter, preferring to leave things to the local Health Authorities. The result of this is that there is wide variation from one area to another, ranging from 10 or more down to 2.7, with the generality being substantially below 6. Since the Report was made, the need for Speech Therapists has been made markedly greater by, for example, the improved treatment of stroke cases, where people now survive who would not have done earlier. A further problem is presented by the release into the community, under recent Health Service rationalisation, of former patients in psychiatric wards, many of whom have severe communication disorders.

Chapter 5

1. A barrister commenting on the case of R has said that he would not

hesitate to sub-poena the other side's expert if he had any reason to believe it would be of advantage to his case. It is possible that this manoeuvre was not available to prosecution counsel in that case, because defence counsel might have not required a written report from his expert, at least on the matter of identification. If that were so, the Cambridge expert did not legally exist, and consequently could not have been the subject of any order. It is possible that the layman will see this as another legalistic dodge to prevent the truth from being heard.

Chapter 6

1. Research is being carried out in the Department of Electronics and Electrical Engineering at UCL, and no doubt in many other institutions, on the use of beams of light instead of electrical impulses in future computers. Another characteristic of light beams, the full implications of which are probably beyond our present understanding, is that they can cross one another without interruption or distortion.
2. Magistrates' courts at present are not permitted to try cases for which a custodial sentence of more than six months could be given.
3. In his Foundation Oration at UCL Union on 22 March 1990, Mr Ludovic Kennedy made some observations on our legal system, many of which are particularly appropriate to this book. I shall quote them without further comment, since they speak clearly enough for themselves:

'... the adversary system of criminal justice which we employ in this country ... is not only extremely childish, but a most unsatisfactory way of attempting to dispense justice. In a situation where one side is doing its best to vanquish the other, truth is apt to fall by the wayside. It is a system ... in which a spurious sense of drama is created which encourages counsel to strike postures and attitudes ... in which counsel see it as one of their tasks to destroy the credibility of the other side's witnesses, whether the issue be pertinent to the verdict or not ... in which some questions that could provide a shortcut to the truth are not allowed to be asked ... in which the evidence of witnesses is shaped by what the prosecution and defence want them to say ... in which other witnesses whose evidence might help shape the jury's verdict are not called for fear of saying the wrong thing ... If we were devising a system of justice today from scratch, would it ever occur to us to dream up something so patently idiotic and inefficient as this?

... the inquisitorial approach has several advantages. Firstly, it avoids the pseudo-dramatic atmosphere of the adversary-system trial ... secondly, the questioning of witnesses in a quiet, firm but non-partisan way is often more productive of a fruitful response ... thirdly, the system saves time for it obviates the need for prosecution and defence to cover ... the same ground ... And lastly, the trial itself does not come grinding to a halt, as so often happens in Britain, when the jury are shuffled out of court so that the judge can decide what is or is not admissible evidence. In a system whose object is to find the truth, there is very little evidence - so long as it is relevant - that is not admissible.

... it is the custom of the court to call as many expert witnesses as the court or counsel may require and by painstaking eliciting of information try, wherever possible, to reach a consensus. This is surely a more effective method of reaching the truth than the adversary approach, which can be both humiliating for the expert witness as well as puzzling for the jury.

... the conviction rate is more than 90% as compared with our conviction rate of only some 50% of contested pleas ...

4. A major advance in international cooperation has been the founding, in recent months, of the International Association for Forensic Phonetics. This arose from the first-ever seminar on the forensic applications of phonetics, organised by Peter French in York in 1989. The IAFP will meet again in 1990. Current membership includes both academics and employees of the judiciary, and draws from several countries, predominantly Great Britain, Germany and the Netherlands. The aims of the IAFP are to establish contacts between individuals and institutions working in the area, and to encourage basic research into relevant aspects of speech.

Bibliography

Abercrombie, D. (1967), *Elements of General Phonetics*, Edinburgh, Edinburgh University Press.

Archbold, (1979) S. Mitchell and J. Huxley Buzzard, (eds), *Pleading, Evidence and Practice in Criminal Cases*, (40th edn) London, Sweet and Maxwell.

Catford, J.C. (1988) *A Practical Introduction to Phonetics*, New York, OUP.

Cross on Evidence (1985) (6th edn) London, Butterworths.

Cruttenden, A. (1986), *Intonation*, Cambridge, Cambridge University Press.

Enderby, P. and Phillip, R. (1986), 'Speech and Language Handicaps: toward knowing the size of the problem', *British Journal of Disorders of Communication*, **21**, pp. 151-165.

Fry, D.B. (1979), *The Physics of Speech*, Cambridge, Cambridge University Press.

Gimson, A.C. (1962), *An Introduction to the Pronunciation of English*, London, Edward Arnold.

Jones, D. (1966), *The Pronunciation of English*, (4th edn) Cambridge, Cambridge University Press.

Kersta, L.G. (1962), 'Voiceprint Identification', *Nature*, (USA). **196**, pp. 1253-1257.

Knowles, G. (1987), *Patterns of Spoken English*, London and New York, Longman.

Künzel, H.J. (1987), *Sprechererkennung*, Heidelberg, Kriminalstik Verlag.

Laver, J. (1980), *The Phonetic Description of Voice Quality*, Cambridge, Cambridge University Press.

Morley, M.E. (1972), *The Development and Disorders of Speech in Childhood*, (3rd edn), Edinburgh and London, Churchill Livingstone.

Nolan, F. and Kniffka, H. (eds) (in press), *Texte zur Theorie und Praxis Forensischer Linguistik*, Tübingen, Max Niemeyer Verlag.

O'Connor, J.D. (1973), *Phonetics*, Harmondsworth, Penguin.

O'Connor, J.D. and Arnold, G.F. (1973) *Intonation of Colloquial English*, (2nd edn), London, Longman.

Phipson on Evidence (1976), (12th edn), London, Sweet & Maxwell.

Pike, K.L. (1943), *Phonetics*, Ann Arbor, University of Michigan Press.

Quirk, R. (1972), *Report on Speech Therapy*, London, HMSO.

Quirk, R., Greenbaum, S., Leech, G. and Svartvik, J. (1985), *A Comprehensive Grammar of the English Language*, London, Longman.

Siebs, T. (1898), *Deutsche Hochsprache*, Berlin.

Selkirk, E.O. (1984), *Phonology and Syntax*, Cambridge, MA., and London, MIT Press.

Sweet, H. (1877), *Handbook of Phonetics*, Oxford, Clarendon Press.

Sweet, H. (1913), *Collected Papers of Henry Sweet*, Oxford, Clarendon Press.

Tosi, O.I. (1979), *Voice Identification: Theory and Legal Applications*, Baltimore, University Park Press.

Wells, J.C. (1982), *Accents of English*, (3 vols), Cambridge, Cambridge University Press.

Index

False conversation 72
Formants 51-53, 56, 57, 59, 61

Goodwin, John 112, 118, 124

Hesitation markers 53, 79

Inquisitorial system 129, 136, 137
Intonation 36-39, 48, 57, 72, 98, 120
Investigative aspects of forensic
  phonetics 64-70

Jury's access to evidence 13

Kennedy, Ludovic (UCL Union
  Foundation Oration 1990) 136,
  137
Krays, The 92-94, 96, 112

Larynx 28, 44
Loudness 29, 41

Nucleus, nuclear tones 38, 39, 51

Oath 12, 122, 134
Objective description of speech 23
Organs of speech 27
Out-of-time cases 88

Phonemic cf phonetic levels of
  analysis 35
Pitch 2, 29, 36-38, 44, 45, 62, 88,
  114, 120
Pitch average 36, 45-48, 57, 97, 98
Pitch range 48, 57
Prejudicial material 13, 14, 105, 106,
  108
Prescriptive approach to phonetics 25,
  135
Problem words 113

Rebuttal evidence 19
Reduction 41, 59
Re-examination 18, 19, 122
Regional accent, *see* Accent
Rhythm 37, 39, 114

Screening of samples for
  discrepancies 88-91
Scretary of State's Tribunal 116,
  117
Segmental units of speech 29-36, 39,
  44, 48, 50, 51, 62, 88, 89, 97, 120
Speaker-identification 3, 4, 7, 8, 20,
  43, 62, 63, 70, 73-91, 107, 109,
  110, 122, 126-128
Speaker-recognition 20, 107, 109, 110,
  111
Spectrogram 8, 50-56, 59
Spectrograph 5
Speech defect 2, 25, 50, 51, 69, 80
Speech Therapist(s) 69, 135
Stammer, *see* Speech defect
Standard pronunciation cf standard
  grammar 25
Stress-timing cf syllable-timing 40
Suppression of relevant evidence 100,
  106, 107, 128, 130, 136
Suprasegmental units of speech 29,
  36-41, 51, 89

Tempo 2
Transcript 42, 70, 76-79
Transcription 76
Trial by combat 16
Trial by expert 17, 132
Trial by jury 18, 131, 132
Trial-within-a-trial 12, 14, 121, 123,
  134

Unintelligible speech 89, 90, 114
Upgraded magistrates' court 131

Variability of speech 2, 3, 5, 90
Vocal cords 44
Vocal tract 28, 29, 34, 57, 126, 127
Vocal-tract print 128
Voice 29
Voice-prints 5, 9, 53, (62), 95, 126,
  128
Voice quality 2, 29, 44, 57, 88, 120

Watergate 71